MAYDAY ON THE MOTHERSHIP

MAYDAY ON THE MOTHERSHIP

Katie O'Toole

Pink Pens Literary House

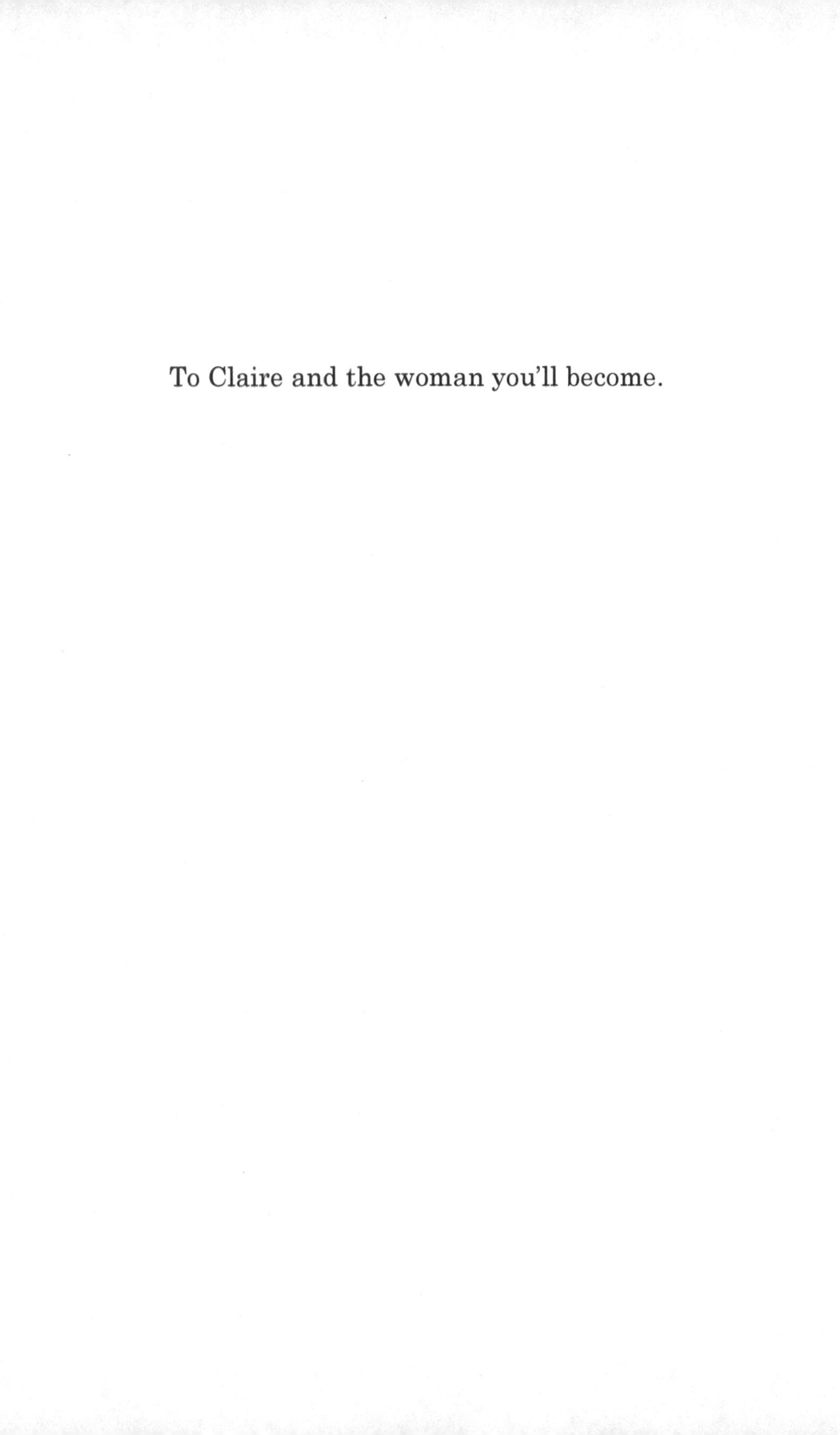
To Claire and the woman you'll become.

Introduction

My daughter's first birthday didn't feel entirely like a celebration. It wasn't only a pink teddy bear themed party for my treasured little girl. It was the anniversary of a death. As I grew lightheaded from blowing up the white balloons covered in little pink ribbon bows, I remembered the woman I was *before*. I didn't want her to return, but I missed her. She was an old friend I'd lost too soon. I wished I could tell her how there was a whole new spectrum of emotion she hadn't even witnessed yet, about the exquisite love she'd feel, and how motherhood would be the odyssey of a lifetime. I'd tell her how she'd be remembered, how I'd tell Claire, our daughter, all about her, and how I loved her. I'd thank her for carrying me here. I'd hug her closely and say goodbye. It had become so clear to me that women shatter and grieve as they become a mother, something new, and even clearer that no one *talks* about it. That's why I wrote this book: to prevent you from feeling blindsided with the slap of each stage of motherhood that will leave you asking, "Am I crazy?" "Is this normal?" "Why hasn't anyone mentioned this?" This book is an honest account, one that I wished women had felt safe enough to share with me.

Postpartum women endure an intense identity crisis, usually in clandestine shame, concealed with smiles and turned attention to the bundle of joy in their arms. Society forgets to lift their gaze from the swaddled baby and perceive the mother too. Through pressured ignominy, society obliges women to feel nothing but gratitude and joy as they lost their body and mind as they knew them. Those beautiful feelings are there too, immensely, but so is the murk. That's the big secret mothers have suppressed for generations, isn't it?

On top of it all, today's women, raised for the corporate machine to be "girl bosses," navigate uncharted expectations in both the household and workplace as mothers. According to Pew Research, (and probably any working woman you'd meet), wives are gaining economic influence while carrying a heavier burden at home. Women match their husbands' income in a third of American households. Our societal structure has been based on the foundation of a nuclear traditional household with a man as the breadwinner and provider. That foundation has now crumbled. As a result, daycares are overflowing. The US Department of Labor states the average daycare cost for just one child ranges from $6,552-$15,600 annually. Business hours and the traditional model of the full-time work week conflict with babies' and postpartum mothers' basic needs. The harsh and inconvenient truth is that American moms are burnt out, and that working full-time *and* being a new mother are in direct odds, at least with the current setup. This book won't convince you that mothers shouldn't work. In fact, I think mothers offer heightened and unmatched skills like patience, compassion, and competence in chaos. In my own career, I've noticed the most talented, organized, creative, hard-working executors of excellence have all been women. I've also seen many of them disappear silently from the workplace as they add "Mother" to their resume. I now know why. I do hope to convince you that we need a change, and it can't be a secret between us gals anymore. I wrote this book to protect you from the loneliness that enveloped me without warning and to open a conversation for evolution toward a more humane world for mothers.

When I realized I was pregnant, I became a sponge. I aimed to soak up every possible drop of information and perspective on the matter. However, in all my maternal studies, I noticed a gap. The choir of available womanly perspectives sounded off, like it was missing a necessary voice. It was that of whom seemed to me like this common modern woman, probably like you and millions of other women out there. The only women I saw sharing their experiences were celebrities and influencers who made their own schedules. Early on, I worried I was already on the verge of postpartum depression, but popular books about it seemed to be *MILF* by British pop star Paloma Faith or *Down Came The Rain* by Brooke Shields. How would a pop star or Brooke fucking Shields understand me? She's Brooke fucking Shields, I thought. I'd be lucky enough to have her eyebrows, let alone her lifestyle as a mother. I found Sarah Hoover's *The Motherload* compelling, but even she was a cool NYC influencer married to a renowned artist, equipped with a night-nanny and freedom of choice to work when she wanted. I loved these books, but I didn't know anyone like this in my "real life," and yet these were the only voices I could find. That's just not the broad story of American Motherhood in the 21st century. I think that's unfair to you and me. There was no blueprint for the style of mothering I had ahead of me. There was no public content for solidarity and relatability, or the knowing that someone would understand and share this holistic load of millions of women in Western culture. I felt more and more alone in the motherhood experience.

- Where were the women like me or like any of my friends and family?
- The women who work truly fulltime jobs with no freedom of schedule?
- The women who are expected to "do it all?" The grown up "girl bosses"
- The women who will only get to see their baby for an hour between work and bedtime and wonder how their babies will even know them as their absent mommy?

There are too many secrets among mothers and the systems stacked against them. We'll cover them together. The biggest one is that women actually *can't* have it all, at least not in the way society demands of them.

Without these accounts and discussions, society will never adjust to meet the needs of modern mothers, and they and their babies will continue to suffer as a result. Women should have freedom to feel it all out loud, honestly with each other and the rest of society. They, their partners, and their employers should be educated and prepared for what they are about to experience so they have the tools and resources that are often life-saving.

The new adolescence

Remember what a wreck you were as a teenager in "adolescence?" Me too. In the 1970s, medical anthropologist, Dana Raphael, coined the term "matrescense," or the "time of mother-becoming." Like adolescence, it refers to one of life's profound metamorphoses, but this time it's heavier than a bad eye shadow look or mouth full of braces. She wrote,

"Childbirth brings about a series of very dramatic changes in the new mother's physical being, in her emotional life, in her status within the group, even in her own female identity."

Matrescence forced me into emotional, social, professional, and medical confrontations I never saw coming. It crushed every part of me. It also molded a new woman whose capacity for love and compassion became immeasurable, uncontainable. Claire's birthday was secretly a birthday of my own too. The weakest parts of me transformed into bold confidence. In my first year as a mother, I gained new interests and passions. I discovered purpose and direction. Creating life with my own body and soul drew me closer to the divine than ever before. I felt otherworldly at times. Motherhood released me from the chains I'd woven tightly around my workplace martyrdom as a working woman and breadwinner. It released me from the stress of tying my self-worth and only living purpose to corporate productivity. I wished I could have seen any of it coming.

Why silence is dangerous

I've wondered how brighter my path may have been had women felt comfortable to share honestly with me and prepare me for what was to come. I had only been told my entire life how wonderful, easy, and beautiful pregnancy and motherhood would be. When I faced much of the opposite instead, I felt like an outsider. I think often about women, trapped in abashment and guilt, who assume they aren't normal and suffer in silence. In 2021, the CDC found 10-20% of all postpartum deaths were related to mental health struggles such as postpartum depression and all its faces. I wondered how this was still the case when motherhood is our most ancient experience as women. This candor and free range to grieve and be reborn is life-or-death.

I heard grief expert David Kessler say on *The Skinny Confidential Him & Her* podcast, "What we run from pursues us." Unhealed motherhood is a dangerous space of fractured identity. Women and families should be allowed face it head on, armored with knowledge and preparation. Too often women are afraid. They fear that, because few can understand or empathize with the pregnancy, birth, and postpartum experience, they'll be seen as insane. They fear being seen as ungrateful or ignoring their privilege of having a healthy baby or surviving the process when others don't.

To women: If you can, involve a mental health professional. Grieve and mourn each version of you unapologetically and loudly. It's the only way to carve room for the new version of you who is born in postpartum. Like your baby, she will be a stranger and scared to arrive here. Welcome her warmly and befriend her. She needs you too.

If nothing else, I hope this book provides you with the confidence to speak up for yourself and your baby at home with your partner, at work with your superiors, and in the hospital room with the medical staff. Let's be honest with each other and the women who will come after us about what we truly experience and *need* as a result. I'm not a doctor offering medical advice, nor a professor writing a textbook, rather a friend inviting you for a glass (a bottle) of wine as we lift the veil and take an honest look at the mess we face. Maybe one day together, we can tidy it up!

1 Losing Identity

"Hurry, let's split this Adderall!" I opened the orange and white capsule and carefully poured the minuscule blue beads evenly into each side like doll-sized shot glasses. I handed one to my best friend Carly. We'd applied the final touches to our makeup, squeezing together in the narrow bathroom mirror of our tiny New York City hotel room overlooking the East Village.

"Cheers to 30, bitch," she said with a clink. We tossed back the mini-goblets of uppers and chased with champagne.

On the way downstairs to meet my girlfriends for my birthday dinner, I admired my reflection in the mirrored elevator walls in my skintight black mini dress. I was the thinnest and healthiest I'd ever been. I felt confident in my body for the first time, and I felt proud to be at my physical peak turning 30. Pregnant me, in puffy physical shambles, reminisced often on this version of me and couldn't believe how quickly she disappeared.

Millennial and Gen Z girls see our bodies through such an unforgiving and dysmorphic lens, don't we? In the era of America's Next Top Model and brutal tabloid covers in the grocery store lines, a wildly critical culture formed our self-images. While my mom loaded the groceries onto the cashier's conveyor belt, I'd read about Jessica Simpson, whom tabloids referred to as "Jumbo Jessica," who looked "beefy" in her size 6 jeans as she raced to "bounce back." Pregnancy changes a woman's body completely. Vainly, I wasn't ready to say goodbye to this reflection.

We celebrated my incoming thirties era with cocktails and Instagram stories, barely touching our entrées and rushing to the club next door. Fueled by adrenaline, Veuve Clicquot, and Adderall, we drank and danced into the morning.

"Well shit, we still fucking got it," my friend Alex jokingly yelled across the lights and music.

This horizon of my thirties exhilarated me. I thought I'd feel defeated about turning 30, unmarried and childless. What I noticed instead is how much I loved this version of myself. I thought she would be boring and old. Instead, she was fun, confident, driven, and successful. She was the woman I imagined as a kid. I knew what she liked to do, eat, drink, buy, and read. At restaurants she'd go right for the Sancerre or Chianti or Chenin Blanc. She'd tried all the wines by now and no longer needed to ask the server what's similar to the cheap red blend she could barely afford at 24. I knew her professional direction. She was in corporate sales and always rose to leadership roles with the corporate ladder in mind. I knew what clothes, colors, and makeup flattered her. I knew who she enjoyed spending time with and reserved time for only them. My days were my own. My body was my own. I'd survived my awkward years of puberty, my teenage years, my twenties, and now I'd made it. I thought I'd always feel like this amazing woman. I had no idea that this would be the last time I'd truly spend with her.

Judgement

New York always reminded me of motherhood because my mom was born in Manhattan, and we'd always seen it as our dream city.

"There's no other place on earth like it," she'd tell me.

I'd worked my ass off since elementary school for this woman I'd become, and New York was the best place to celebrate her arrival. I imagined taking my mom's soul with me. I did this for us, I said internally as I landed at JFK, wishing it was a mother-daughter trip.

On the flight, I thought about how I'd probably be a mom in the next year or two. I dreamed of holding a precious little baby in my arms. However, along with these fuzzy feelings, I also feared the judgement pregnancy brings upon women. When girls hit child-bearing age, suddenly, we're monitored closely. Society watches girls to see if they can maintain purity, waiting for them to slip up at every step. For women, teenage pregnancy is one of the most damning cultural mores. Young women face immense scrutiny and judgement. We live in fear of getting pregnant, and I think it leaves a scar as we aim to start a family, even on purpose, later in life.

Looking down at the tiny buildings from the airplane window, I thought about my own biological grandmother down there in New York decades ago. I imagined the pressure she felt as an unwed mother, and how she gave my mom to her family members to adopt. I wondered why, even today, our culture hadn't evolved much more. Today's women *still* face a similar magnifying glass, and I knew I'd soon be under it too.

Home Sweet Home

I nursed my NY hangover in the little white house I grew up in in Pittsburgh. My mom grew up there too. It wasn't just a house. It was an atrium of my heart with its pink and green stained-glass windows and white Victorian woodwork.

"They don't make houses like this anymore," everyone commented upon entering.

Stepping off the bucolic front-porch, the living room greeted you from the front door with high ceilings and built-in bookcases with a wide mantel, leading to the dining room adorned with two while pillars and an antique gold and crystal chandelier. Although it was small, it was a work of art and craftsmanship. If you didn't look too closely, you wouldn't notice the tilting foundation or chips in the wood molding.

As I walked through my routines, I was welcomed by memories of where my mother hugged me for extra-long one day after school in the dining room, where we cried together in what was once her bedroom, where I watched movies with her in the living room, where she held me and prayed with me at night in what was my childhood bedroom. I'd stare at the ceiling at night and remember her tickling my arm while I fell asleep. As I made my morning coffee, I'd admire the brown wooden cabinets my dad installed as a surprise for my mom in the 90s. He's a tough, Irish, blue-collared man who expressed his love through home improvement projects. She came back from a trip to visit her college friend to a brand-new kitchen, handcrafted by her loving husband. Although I'd painted the walls a modern eggshell and updated the hardware, the cabinets were the same, and they were a keepsake of their love. I tied my shoes on the antique rocking chair in the living room where my nana rocked my mom as a baby, and she rocked me. I imagined I'd rock my own baby in that same chair one day. I could still hear my mom's voice and feel her there. She died when I was 17 from breast cancer, and it became an emotional time capsule. I imagined, even if I were stuck earthbound as a ghost, no doubt it's where I'd haunt. It was all part of me and epitomized "home."

I didn't know how I'd move one day, but I knew I'd need to in order to become a mother. It was so old. Everything needed to be replaced and not the fun aesthetic stuff. I mean the roof, the sewer, and the electrical. It seemed irresponsible to stay much longer. Opening the chapter of motherhood meant closing all the chapters I'd spent there all at once. The stories of my grandparents raising their family there, my childhood, my single years living alone and painting the front door pink, and now this life with my boyfriend, Connor. You'll meet him soon. I dreaded the inevitable losses every time a shingle fell off and dreaded motherhood a bit too as a result, but I basked in its comfort for now.

When I got pregnant, I accepted that my home, which I considered another facet of my identity, would have to go as I created a *new* home.

Connor

Connor and I squeezed into that little house with our two dogs. They shared many of Connor's same qualities— large, loud, and messy. I'd chase all three of them around lovingly with a Mr. Clean Magic Eraser, never able to keep up. Taz is an oversized chocolate lab who weighs more than I do. Punkin is a stubborn and rambunctious English bulldog, also oversized and usually covered in mud and slobber.

As a couple, Connor and I were serious, but I didn't have a ring yet. I felt that pressure. He didn't. "I'm marrying you one day. What's the rush?"

At 29, I finally started to clap back with, "My biological clock!!"

We'd been together for a little over three years, and I'd known him through mutual friends for closer to a decade. I knew he was someone I'd be with for the long haul, but I craved the show of commitment. I noticed every hand of almost every woman my age scintillating with an icy rock that said, "Look, a boy picked me!" My naked left finger seemed to scream, "Look at me, no one wanted me!" It mimicked the sunken feeling in my chest when no one asked me to Homecoming in high school. "It's because we're fat, isn't it?" asked that chubby 12-year-old inside me.

For Connor, being in love and having fun was enough for now. He's very type B, my opposite. He's captivating and changes the energy when he walks in the room. Physically, you can't miss him with his broad chest and fiery red beard, but you'll hear his loud deep voice making someone laugh before you see him. Everything about him is larger than life.

"We might like him better than you," my sisters joked when they met him.

He bursts every thought and feeling outward. It's an honest quality, and it's necessary to pull communication out of me sometimes. Our opposing communication styles made for tortuous conflict, though, usually ending in a repetitive stalemate. We'd each stew for a few days, accept that we won't understand each other, and just pretend it didn't happen, buying the other a snack from the gas station as an olive branch. Parenthood would later highlight how important healthier conflict habits are to a couple. Nothing tests a couple like becoming parents. After we had our daughter, I looked back on this version of us and wished we knew what we were about to tackle so that we could have prepared our relationship to better weather the hurricane of parenthood.

"He has a good heart," Carly would remind me whenever I was mad at him. She was right. I was in love with him. I could see the future dad in him. He made everyone in the room feel safe. He was a good masculine mix of passionate, sturdy, and bold, yet still tender and loving.

Let's hold onto these good qualities for later chapters because you'll be mad at him.

2 The Ticking Clock

"I'm getting you pregnant when you get back from New York," Connor said point-blank at the dinner table. My eyes widened looking down at the white tablecloth.

I reached for my glass of chianti. "Okay," I said, not sure if he was serious.

We were eating at one of our favorite local Italian restaurants, Alla Famiglia. It has an old charm feel to it and the vodka pasta is to die for. Going to restaurants was a love language of sorts. We'd spontaneously text each other saying, "We have reservations this Friday at 8PM," for a surprise dinner date. It was at these dinner tables that we'd discuss real-life stuff, lubricated to cover the tough subjects of our relationship by a bottle of wine. After I'd enlightened him about my biological clock, we decided we didn't want to ruin the fun of planning our wedding by tying it to the same anxiety-driven deadlines of the need to have a baby.

"I'm serious. Why not just get pregnant now and married later? It's not the *right* way, but it can be our way." He pushed aside the calamari and reached for my hand across the table. This did feel like it lifted some of the pressure I'd been feeling all these years.

I returned his smile, "Okay. Why not?"

I'd first heard the clock ticking when I turned 25. It started softly but surely. I was enjoying being single, but the math kept me up at night…

"If I meet someone now… we'll date for a few years… get engaged… be engaged for a year, plan a wedding… get married… be married for a year or two, and before you know it, I'm 32 and limited on how many kids I can even have at all," I spiraled, staring at my ceiling. "Who knows what my fertility would look like by then…"

I know that women can and do have babies late in life. It would make sense to do it later since I'd probably be more mentally and financially ready to be a parent, but I just didn't love that idea for myself. Age 35 means medically a "high-risk" pregnancy and birth. The medical term is literally a "geriatric" pregnancy. After 30, and especially after 35, women have higher risk for miscarriage, gestational diabetes, preeclampsia, and delivery complications. The baby is at higher risk for birth defects and chromosome abnormalities too. That's *if* women can even get pregnant with declining fertility as we age. A study by The University of St. Andrews and Edinburgh University had recently found that women lose 90% of their eggs by 30 years old. Only 3% of their eggs remained at 40. I already knew too many women who'd hit the mid-thirties and found they'd waited too long and couldn't afford IVF treatments. The US Department of Health & Human Services estimates the cost for a single cycle of IVF to range from $15,000-$20,000, and it's not guaranteed to work.

Stats like these haunted me, and I knew I wasn't alone. "Haunt" seems to be the right word here because I'd even seen a horror movie on Hulu about it called *Clock.* The main character's time on her biological clock is running out, and the pressure from family, friends, and society manifests in ghostly apparitions that psychologically torment her.

My mind raced like this for years, and I tried to get Connor's mind to keep up the pace. I envied men and their ability to conceive well into an elderly state if they wanted

to. Remember when Al Pacino had a baby at 83 with his
29-year-old girlfriend? I imagined Connor one day deciding
that I'd expired and wanting someone younger with fresher
eggs. It's just not something that many men think about the
way women do. When we first started dating in our
twenties, I once overheard Connor in conversation at a
backyard bonfire party.

"I can probably see myself having kids in my early
fifties. That's the goal," he said with a swig of his beer met
with agreeing nods from the other guys. He wasn't alone in
the sentiment.

I'd read an NPR article on the subject. The headline
read, "Fatherhood at 40? It's Becoming a Lot More
Common." Studies had found that twice as many dads of
newborns are now in the 40+ age group, compared to the
1970's. Men do have somewhat of a clock, as sperm
quantity and quality decrease after 40, but it's still not as
finite as it is for women. I stewed in the unfairness that it's
possible for men like Connor to have babies whenever they
please.

The next day, I was in the shower, and he was sitting
on the bathroom floor to be close to me. He never wanted
to be apart. If we didn't shower together, he would at least
stay in the room. Even when I'd pee, I'd have to lock the
door or else he'd come in saying "I miss you!" No one,
aside from my parents, had ever loved me like he did. Still,
I was nervous to have the kids conversation.

I lathered shampoo into my hair and tried my best to
casually bring it up. "You know how you were saying last
night that you want to have kids in your fifties?"

"Yeah, what about it? That'll just be such a perfect age.
I can enjoy my 30s and 40s, traveling and who knows what
else. It would give me more time to make the money I'd

like to have by then too," he said, breaking my heart with each word as he packed weed into his little green bowl pipe.

"Okay that makes sense. I do want you to realize, though, that it will mean you'll have to have those kids with someone else." I tried to gently steer his logic. "We won't be able to be together long-term. Do you realize that?"

"What do you mean?" he said flicking on the lighter.

My tone was no longer cool and collected. "Cool girl" had left the conversation.

"Connor, women can't have babies in their fifties. *I* cannot have babies in my fifties, and we're basically the same age. You will be having those babies later in life with some fucking twenty-five-year-old girl," I said snatching the pipe out of his hand and taking a drag. "How do you not realize this?"

"Oh shit. I mean, I knew that. I guess I just never thought about it," he said so lightly it made my blood boil. This was all just light conversation for him while my future was crumbling.

"This is something we need to figure out. I know that I want to be a mom. You have every right to want babies later in life but, remember, it won't be with me. My clock is ticking. I'll be 30 in a few years, so if you don't see yourself with me long-term like that, please don't waste my time."

He put the bowl down and rolled his eyes as my monologue continued.

"I mean, please don't waste my like… child-rearing years," I pressed.

I probably looked as crazed as my tone, soaking wet with mascara all over my eyes and shampoo suds in my hair.

"Oh my God. Now I'm wasting your time? How did we get here? For Christ's sake, Katie. I was drunk at a party and just said that in conversation not even thinking about it. You're majorly overacting," he said.

"I get that, but Connor this is serious and important to me. What if we stay together for another 3 years and you decide you no longer want to be together and then I'm now left in the dust with old shriveled-up eggs and can't have a baby ever. My life-long dream of being a mom would be gone. Do you understand why this freaks me the fuck out?"

I was embarrassed by my anxious display, so I never brought it up directly again. As the years progressed, so did my anxiety, but he started to affirm that he did want babies with me, and not the younger girl in his fifties. He'd say things like, "when we have our kids…" The comments relieved me a little, but they didn't stop time. The older I got, the louder the ticking grew. By my late twenties, the noise had drowned out, for me, any other goals we had as a couple. As the deadlines approached, Connor must have heard the ticking too because he seemed more ready than I was. By the time I returned from my NYC birthday trip, he was antsy and excited to start a family. My turning 30 was a crescendo for both of us. It was decided.

3 Woman of The House

Despite the clock, counting down like the end of a close football game, I didn't want to feel like we were "trying." That word conjured images of women tracking schedules, taking their temperature, injecting hormones, and forcing sex as a transaction. The Center for Disease Control had tracked declining fertility in the US for years, and federal data would later show in 2025 that the US had its lowest birth recorded at 1.6 children per woman. According to World Bank Data, fertility and birth rates have steadily declined for the last few decades across Europe too. It seemed scary, and I didn't want the pressure. Work was stressful enough, and I wanted to start my family on a peaceful note. Shouldn't having a baby be magic anyway?

I don't know that any woman really is ready to uproot their life in such a way, but *tick tock...*

Connor was ready and excited to be a dad, probably because very little changes for the man in these situations. He envisioned the cute baby giggles and fun memories ahead. He saw taking his son to his first NFL game or tossing a football in the yard. I saw versions of my own future memories too, but I knew the real responsibility of holding down the fort would fall on me. I was afraid this would turn into another household project for me to manage because, like many women, I carried the mental load in our household. My own motherly daydreams competed with worries of rising daycare costs, the effect on my sales career that paid half of our bills, not to mention the toll on my body and mental health. My thin and healthy figure that I'd just made peace with after 30 years would change drastically. I'd say goodbye to my house...THE house. It seemed the sacrificial list went on infinitely for women but was so short for men. The stark contrast pissed me off.

Weaponized Incompetence

When a woman agrees to marriage these days, it appeared that she signs up to be everything all at once; a breadwinner at work, a loving and present mother, fulltime maid, and chef at home with a hot dinner on the table at 5PM sharp. It all better be done gorgeously for social media too. I occasionally noticed women my age on TikTok crying out into the void of the algorithm looking for solidarity with other women battling what therapists now call "weaponized incompetence." *Psychology Today* defines it as "strategically avoiding responsibility by pretending to be incapable or inept at a task so that someone else does it." It's a common theme in modern American households: The wife and mother not only make half the money or more, but they also cook, clean, and overall manage the household, all on top of child-rearing. When she asks a man to do a simple task around the house like laundry or cleaning the bathroom her husband will do it but do it terribly. She'll never ask him again because she knows it won't be done well, and so, most tasks slowly fall on her.

There had been numerous studies analyzing this growing trend for modern women. A Harvard study found that American women handle the majority of the physical *and* mental load of American households. A UCLA study found that a messy house spikes women's Cortisol levels, but not men's. It's not only American homes. The 2023 review of Economics of the Household studied thousands of couples in the UK. The data showed British women spend 10 more hours a week on household chores than men. I read an NPR article in 2023 that opened with, "Women are bringing home the bacon and frying it up too." I already was the maid, chef, breadwinner, homeowner, finance manager, property manager, handyman, interior decorator, party planner, calendar manager, and now, I'd have to be the mother too? It seemed to be the biggest role of all.

Connor would have to completely change for us, and I didn't know how to convince him to do it.

I saw a movie about this called *Tully,* starring Charlize Theron. It features a stay-at-home mother of three, her husband, and her night-nanny. The movie ends with a twist that the night-nanny we'd gotten to know throughout the movie had actually been the mother's hallucination. In a state of extreme sleep deprivation and physical and mental exhaustion, her brain created this night-nanny as a coping mechanism. Her husband was checked out and focused on his own life, work, hobbies, meals, and sleep. Although he loved them, his life wasn't affected much by having children, whereas his wife's life turned upside down. The character demonstrates how motherhood, especially with an unsupportive partner, can entirely deplete a woman. It can utterly delete the person she was physically, mentally, professionally, and emotionally. In one scene, the very pregnant main character is at her wits end. She walks into a coffee shop for a treat to pick up her spirits, as one does. After a judgmental Karen reminds her pregnant woman shouldn't drink coffee, she sits down to sulk into a muffin and latte. A woman approaches her table whom we learn was her former roommate from years ago, a past life. The woman was thin, bright, clearly healthy, and well-dressed, what the mother used to be too. The scene illustrates the grim dissimilarity of who this mother could have still been had she not been eaten alive by motherhood and marriage. She'd turned into a fat, tired, uninspired, and depressed shell of herself. The story climaxes with a car accident and another scene that disturbed me. The wife was in a state of postpartum delirium with no help from her husband. He stood clueless in the bustling hospital hallway in the ER to discuss his wife's prognosis. I recognized him as the same actor as Berger from *Sex & The City*, a character I already hated.

"Her brother sprang for a night-nanny, so she's getting help, she's getting sleep…" her husband said like a confused child.

"Actually, we think she's experiencing extreme exhaustion and sleep deprivation," the doctor interrupted him, with a furrowed brow and a look of serious concern.

"I don't know how. It seems like she's better than she's ever been. I guess there's been a couple moments that have been out of character…uh," he stammered. "But I wouldn't ever expect her to drive drunk like that, you know, or leave the house without telling me so no one's watching the kids."

"But weren't you home?" The doctor asked rhetorically. It never occurred to him that he could be watching his own children.

Doesn't it seem that moms can't win these days? We're expected to fit the old-school trad wife persona: a soft and present mom who lives only to serve her children and husband. Yet even the girls embracing that lifestyle receive societal backlash for succumbing to patriarchal pressures our gender just recently defeated. Lest we forget American women couldn't control their own finances until the 1970s. *Vogue, The New Yorker,* and many others have published articles criticizing tradwives. Society isn't happy with us as the stay-at-home mom anymore, but they're also not happy with us as the breadwinner either. We don't fit into the home comfortably anymore. Where do we go? The answer seems to be a new form of woman, somewhere in the middle, but societal structures don't seem ready for her.

Fulfilling my own dream of motherhood would come at immense cost, and it scared me. I was in such a rush all these years leading up to 30, but now that I finally had the opportunity to start a family, I wasn't sure I was ready, and neither was the world around me.

4 Working Mother

As a little girl, I played with baby dolls, shushing and comforting them while I cooked sticks and leaves on my pink Fisher Price play-kitchen on our front porch. My friends and I would put our rubber sparkly kickballs under our shirts to pretend to be pregnant and play "house" constantly. My career had shoved that version of me down deep. I'd become a cold corporate control freak to survive the modern necessity of womanhood, but I'd always been the soft motherly type at my core, or at least I wanted to be. I was in corporate sales. I loved it, but it was high-stress and unpredictable. I spent 10 hours a day negotiating deals with mean finance guys and eye-rolling HR directors. Urgency was key to beating the competition. I put in early mornings and late nights. I reminded myself often of Martha Stewart's comment to Betheny Frankel on The Apprentice, "Women in business don't cry." I left all emotion at home and came to work with armor, ready to match anyone's energy and win the deal. I thanked God daily for my friends at work to lighten my mood.

As I considered being a mom, I missed that little girl in her play-kitchen and apologized to her that I somehow screwed up along the way and missed the opportunity for the soft life we'd dreamed of. I no longer felt right in my place in society. I didn't seem to fit anywhere.

Motherhood in Previous Generations

I looked up to my mom as a child, but I now realized I wouldn't get to be the same type of mother she was. Before she had me, she was a social worker. She was compassionate and saintly. She volunteered with the poor in her spare time and did the same professionally. I once found photos she'd taken in the 70s and 80s of dirt-covered children in rags. A shack made of broken wood stood behind them. When I asked about the pictures, she explained she used to organize groups of volunteers to help people in Appalachia who in some areas lived in extreme poverty. She'd teach them to read and bring them clothes and food.

"Why don't you do that anymore?" I remember asking her.

"I spend all my time with you now," she said with a kiss.

Data from Pew Research Center showed that, for my mom's generation, nearly half of American women were stay-at-home moms with a husband-provider. In 2012, that dropped to 20%. Today, many women risk their health to return to work right away, likely out of financial dependency on the paycheck. In 2012, Department of Labor studies showed that one in four working moms returned to work just two weeks after birth. No wonder our birth rates are dropping.

Through her career, my mom was passionate and influential in so many lives. It was important work, but she quit her career cold-turkey when she got pregnant with me and became a stay-at-home mom, as many women in her generation and the generations before that did. I became the recipient of all that generosity, passion, and selflessness, but I always wondered if she missed her old life before I became the center of it. She'd never have admitted it if she did.

She parented me with that same empathetic and kind approach and always taught me to help others in need, even when we were in need ourselves. Every Christmas season, she'd take me up to the front of Church to the "Angel Tree," a tree filled with pieces of paper with first names of children in need in our community. One Christmas when I was about eight, I excitedly picked a name that said "Katie." I daydreamed about who this poor little girl with the same name as me might be. Maybe she was blonde and went to the school across the street from mine. I bet she liked makeup and Barbies like I did. My mom took me to the mall and let me pick out a shimmery butterfly-shaped velvet box with kid-friendly makeup inside. "She's going to love it," I squealed. We wrapped it and put it under the tree with a prayer for Katie and her family to have a Merry Christmas. On Christmas Eve that week, a knock came to our door. It was a woman from our church.

"Hello and Merry Christmas!" she said with a smile and an armful of gift-wrapped boxes.

I was hiding behind the pillar in our dining room. My mother whispered with her at the door, but I could hear them.

"An anonymous 'angel' from our church wanted your daughter Katie to have a Merry Christmas and someone bought her this gift," the woman said proudly, thinking my mom would be overjoyed and grateful.

She recognized the pink wrapping and started to cry. It was our gift. Someone in our church knew my parents were struggling with my mom being sick. I got to keep the butterfly box, and I realized the Katie was me. I learned then that my mother always poured from an empty cup for others this way and even more so for me. I wanted to be the same kind of person and mom one day.

That type of mother is selfless and 100% present. She picked me up from school every day at 2:30PM sharp with a huge smile that I could see all the way through the parking lot in the windshield. I'd get in the car greeted with nothing but her sweet, soft voice.

"Hi sweetheart, what did you learn today?" The radio was off because she wanted to hear every detail. She was all ears and hung on every word.

She was there for every cheerleading practice at 3PM, every presentation mid-morning, and she was there to drop off my lunch I'd forgotten or to pick me up when I felt sick. There were no constraints of "business hours." There was no delineation of when she was allowed to be a mom. She was a mom all the time. I'd begun to realize I wouldn't get to do the same.

The impossibly modern "Working Mom"

As I reflected on my mom's parenting style, my mind rushed forward to *my* future child's day. 2:30 PM was during prime business hours, and I wouldn't be off work to pick them up from school. I wouldn't get to drop them off in the morning either because I needed to be at work at 7:30 AM, *maybe* 7:45 AM at the latest, and the day ended at 5:00 PM with a commute thereafter. I wouldn't be there for science fairs, presentations, or cheerleading practice. I remembered that even Trick-Or-Treating in our city began at 5:00 PM and ended at 7:00 PM. It seemed that moms who work fulltime just don't get to participate in these things. Like most corporate employees, I barely made it home before 6:30 PM each day. I had nothing to left to give in my day-to-day schedule, and for the first time, at 30, it broke my heart.

What if my child was sick, I wondered. Elena Bridgers has a Substack series called, "Motherhood Until Yesterday," and she recently pointed out, "Households with 2+ kids are sick 56% of the year, but Americans only get 5 total sick days if they're lucky."

This is especially an issue for those with infants. A common cold for you and me as adults can be very serious and life-threatening for an infant. The mother is an infant's immune system for the first 6 months of life via breastmilk and physical contact. (We'll talk more about that later.) How can we rip them apart like this?

The corporate world as we know it doesn't account for parenthood. It was clear to me that it needed to change, but it only seemed clear to people who were *already* mothers. Since women are so tight-lipped about the mother-becoming experience, this major human issue doesn't cross the minds of employers or colleagues.

How many women like my mom even exist anymore? I wondered. I know they're out there, but no wonder the number seemed to be dwindling. I knew stay-at-home-moms still existed, but it only seemed possible for the wealthy or those who don't make enough money to outweigh childcare costs.

The Girl Boss Factory

My generation was groomed for this corporate machine. We weren't taught to make room for being a mom in our futures. We grew up hearing terms like "girl boss," and "girl power." Until this recent generation, schools raised kids for both the office and the home. "Home

Economics" classes used to be a staple of American high school curriculum, beginning in the late 1800s. Students, mostly the girls, learned about cooking, sewing, and childcare. Now, barely any schools offer these courses. Instead, our generation of little girls mastered Microsoft PowerPoints and Excel spreadsheets that we'd soon need to produce in the corporate world for 9-10 hours a day. It seemed to be the only natural option and the only respected goal. Since the 90's, women have been surpassing men in achieving a Bachelor's Degree year after year. Career success is now the only focus. Get good grades so that you can get into a good college so that you can get a good fulltime job and make money… The plan stopped there.

Grown-ups constantly asked us as kids, "What do you want to be when you grow up?" We didn't know that suddenly as we approached our 30s, the follow-up questions would become, "Do you also want to be a mom?" "How will you do both?"

I only personally knew one stay-at-home-mom my age. She quit her career with her second pregnancy, this time with twins. Her fulltime work schedule wouldn't allow her the time off to care for two premature twins and a toddler. She and her husband tried to make it work but quickly had to sell their house and move back in with their parents, unable to keep up with today's economic demands on one income. This is a common struggle for the middle class right now, and again, since no one talks to us about this, it comes without warning.

"We couldn't afford daycare for three kids but couldn't afford to do it all on one income either," she told me.

For the middle class, even upper-middle class, there seems to be no easy setup on a single income. It seemed only the rich got to choose. I secretly started to resent

Connor for not being wealthy enough to comfortably support the lifestyle I suddenly dreamed of. I hated that we were just *normal.* I'd watch videos on social media of Pookie and Jet, influencers who'd become famous from their wholesome yet lavish lifestyle. Pookie was a stay-at-home wife and Jet catered to her every wish. He brought her breakfast in bed every Sunday and showered her in Hermes gifts. I imagined that she must be so excited to be a mom, stress-free.

When I walked in the door at the end of my workday, I was exhausted and still pissed off about the finance guy who belittled me or the contractor who screamed at me over the phone that day. I was still emotionless, cold, and guarded as I kicked off my heels, already game-planning for tomorrow. I'd usually smoke a joint with Connor just to calm my nervous system enough to be a present girlfriend in the evenings, let alone a mother.

How could I so quickly change, the second my key entered the front door, into that soft and loving mom inside me, just to quickly chain her up again by 7AM the next morning?

Modern motherhood didn't look very appetizing, yet I craved it deeply.

5 Probably Pregnant

I closed out the best 30th birthday month with a crowded Halloween house party at my friend Natalie's place. Connor and I dressed up as Chuckie and Chuckie's bride. I planned our costumes for weeks, down to detailed purple and red shading on the makeup scars on his head. The party was packed, loud, and decorated to the nines with skeletons and spider webs. This was our lively group of friends who love to party and stay out all night. They're a blast. I took an Adderall someone handed me and ate way too many red Jell-O shots. Everyone there was between 23 to 33, a polarizing age group especially in women. One was engaged and just bought a new home, while another offered me a line of coke, another still lived with her parents, another just bought her second house. Barely anyone in our friend group, though, was ready to have kids yet, so we kept our baby-wish to ourselves. We had a few friends from college who did have kids, but we rarely saw them anymore. They'd never be out this late.

Hammered and having a blast, we headed to an after-hours club downtown and went home still wired around 4AM. We had drunk sex still partially in our costumes and I fell asleep smiling. We slept in until 9AM, took our time waking up with the dogs, and went to our favorite coffee shop for cinnamon lattes the next morning. It was a typical weekend morning together, and I wouldn't notice the freedom of it until we no longer had it as parents. We didn't think about the pregnancy when we had sex, but the difference was, we'd stopped trying *not* to get pregnant.

A few weeks later, I was taking a walk in Florida, keeping an eye out for the neighborhood alligator. I was in town to visit my dad and stepmom, Sandy, for Thanksgiving. I was in shape, but I felt unusually tired. Must be all the travel, I thought. I called Rachael, another one of my best friends, to chat with. She sat behind me in Mr. Jackson's Algebra class, and we bonded over our confusion. We've talked on the phone almost daily ever since. At 30, I started to notice the differences in our lifestyles and what it would mean for our futures as women and mothers.

The Modern Fairytale

Rachael used to be a cog in a corporate machine like me. When she met her now husband, he quickly offered to have her quit her 9 to 5 and move out of state with him to support her small business endeavors. I wished someone could whisk me away from the corporate life too. That seemed to be the modern princess fairytale. Being "swept off your feet" these days meant being swept into unemployment or self-employment bliss with the freedom to be a mother. Whenever I was ready to have a baby, I wanted a man to rescue me out of my career-life so that I'd have time to be a mom. I never felt this before. I used to love having a career. I enjoyed the dignity of working to put food on my own table. I cherished the freedom of not needing to depend on a man or anyone to financially support myself. It all changed as I approached motherhood. Every "girl boss" bone in my body had started to crumble. Rachael was an example of the type of woman I now wanted to be. She still worked very hard but made her own schedule and had freedom of time and choice.

"What are you up to?" She'll say as she calls me at 2PM EST on a Wednesday.

"I'm working, bitch," I reply, shackled to my computer counting down the minutes until 5:00PM.

If she wanted to attend a Pilates class or take a walk, go on a trip on a whim, she could align it with her work at her own pace. Even things like a doctor's appointment or running to the post office that needed to happen during business hours sent me into a spiral. Becoming a mom only emphasized this more. What about OB appointments, pediatrician appointments, school plays, soccer games… Freedom of time. That, to me, is wealth.

Sixty hours a week went to my job and its demands. There's a reason they call it working "fulltime."

I worried, where would a baby fit into this lifestyle?

Help! I've fallen pregnant & I can't get up!

"I'm hopping in the shower. I'll be right out to help you cook," I yelled to Sandy after my walk.

I stepped over the tub to get out of the shower in the steamy bathroom. I suddenly lost feeling and strength in my right leg. It felt like a heavy log, and I fell on the tile floor with a thud. I'd later learn limb weakness can be common in pregnancy.

"Are you okay honey?" Sandy yelled from the kitchen.

"Yeah, sorry I just dropped something!" I didn't want to worry them.

I wasn't hurt, but what the hell was that? Maybe I overdid it on my walk? The humidity? Something was off in my body. I sipped my wine and stirred the gravy that I'd turned into a cauldron of clumps. The Thanksgiving food grossed me out, and I didn't have an appetite. I wouldn't dare say it out loud. Food aversion…Another pregnancy symptom I'd never heard of before.

I poured the rest of my wine down the sink, remembering that Connor hadn't been pulling out anymore. Could this really be it?

"I'm turning in early tonight. You guys have fun! Goodnight! Love you," I hugged my dad after dinner, barely keeping my eyes open.

The next morning, I just knew. I wasn't even late yet, but I felt something inside me as if a little marble appeared in what I assumed could only be my uterus. I was never aware of my organs in my body before, but there was my uterus, and I was pregnant. I knew it.

I'll take a test at the airport as soon as I'm alone, I thought, as I tried to act natural stirring my morning coffee on the couch with Sandy. That Halloween party night… did we really conceive dressed as chuckie and chuckie's bride? I cringed, petting Ralphie on my lap.

As I sat there internally panicking, in some odd circumstance of divine timing, my friend Alex texted me.

"I THINK I'M FUCKING PREGNANT."

I texted back, "What's going on?? Did you take a test??

"Not yet but I'm about to, and I'm freaking out."

"OMG. Okay also…Dude me too…"

"OMG."

I know it was a bit strange that I told her before Connor or my family, but I needed to vent, and I wasn't ready to announce anything. I think it's unfair to expect women to keep such a big secret and carry the weight alone for a while, and plus, I wasn't even sure it was real yet.

6 Anticipation

Never again will I fly during Thanksgiving weekend. I had a delay that made me miss my layover, and by this point, it was late at night, and I was so tired. The Dunkin Donuts, one of the only businesses in the small Melbourne, FL airport, was out of Donuts. Depravity. Flights were cancelled all over. It was crowded mayhem. Usually, this airport was empty and chill with a few people drinking beer at the little tiki bar in the middle of the terminal. Tonight, the staff handed out beers and pop cans at the gates to try to appease the people who'd been sitting there all day and night with one delay after another.

Finally, after hours of waiting, I got a flight connecting in ATL. I'm there all the time for work, so I knew the airport well. This time was different. Apocalyptic crowds were shoulder to shoulder everywhere. People were yelling and pushing as I peeled my heavy eyes open looking for a store. I needed a pregnancy test, but it was so late that everything was closed. Plus, I needed to hurry to the airport hotel to hopefully get three hours of sleep before my new flight back to Pittsburgh… I had to work in about eight hours. The trains were so packed I couldn't get close, so I walked for an hour to baggage claim and then Ubered to the hotel. My body felt like it was breaking down, and the probable pregnancy seemed all the more real.

Exhaustion outweighed suspense for now. I have to get to work. I'm out of PTO days, I thought.

"I'm sorry baby," I gently touched my lower belly and imagined who could be in there.

I felt so guilty that, if I was really pregnant, I was treating this baby this way when its life was so delicate. This wasn't the calm, healthy, and peaceful body this baby deserved to begin life within. I dreaded a packed day of meetings. I thought about asking for a sick day, but that wouldn't be a good look after the Thanksgiving PTO I just took. Days off were never truly "off" anyway. I knew my phone would ring constantly. I was in sales, and every hour I wasn't seated in front of my laptop meant I wasn't making money toward our livelihood.

Could we afford a baby? Can anyone?

Connor worked just as hard and made about the same money. He's a home renovation plumber, and we both made six figures. It's much more than most in our generation. Many couples our age live paycheck to paycheck. I was grateful for our income, but it never felt like enough. The money funneled right to student loans, car payments, real estate taxes, household repairs, utilities and minor savings. We lived comfortably but still had the inevitable property disaster like our aging roof and sewer looming. God forbid one of us needed dental work or Punkin needed another surgery from swallowing a toy. Like many our age, we were one financial emergency away from major debt. Quitting my job to become a full-time mother wasn't on the table, and I was just now facing it. These anxious thoughts lulled me to sleep in the hotel.

I blinked, and it was time to head back to ATL TSA at 4AM Monday morning. I fought for a spot on the hotel shuttle, waited in a 3-hour security line, and made my flight just in time, out of breath from sprinting through the terminal, more exhausted and cramping like crazy. I

wondered, am I getting my period and I've gotten myself
all worked up for nothing? I bought the in-air Wi-Fi and
googled my symptoms on the plane. I discovered
"implantation cramping." The uterus feels crampy like
menstrual pain as the embryo implants itself to the uterine
wall. I'd never heard of this. I still worried, is this normal,
or had I run my body so ragged that something was wrong
with this baby I haven't confirmed even exists yet?

I rushed home from the airport and ran into the house
with my coat and yesterday's makeup still on, logged
straight onto my laptop to the sound of the Microsoft
Teams jingle signaling the start of a meeting. I took a deep
breath and the workday began. I was locked in for the next
10 hours. Still no test. No time.

As I'd feared, there were no open slots on my Outlook
calendar to be pregnant.

Testing

Finally, after 5, and I had my first moment to breathe. I
just wanted to go to sleep. The low light of our Christmas
decorations we'd put up the week before made the perfect
ambiance for a nap. I missed being a kid on Christmas
break without all this grownup pressure. Most of all, I think
I missed naps. I ordered a test on GoPuff, four of them,
actually.

I'd been there before. We all have, right? We've all sat
quietly in a bathroom studying a white stick at some point.
Emotions are high, no matter which outcome we anticipate.
The three minutes of staring and waiting for the results to
appear, this time, felt strange. In the past when I'd taken
pregnancy tests in my early twenties, I sat there on the
toilet in a panic, praying for a negative. My family would

kill me, I'd be homeless, unemployed, wasted hundreds of thousands on student loans, and my life would be over, I'd think.

I found it jarring how that vision was supposed to change so drastically for women from sheer panic to gratitude. As girls grow into adulthood, pregnancy starts out as the biggest fear and shame you could bring upon your family as a teenager and young adult. We fervently avoid it and fear the judgement that comes with it. Then, BOOM! Suddenly, you're 30, and it's the greatest gift! A blessing! What a mindfuck, I thought.

I still felt like that nervous 19-year-old on the toilet. I was still her, just with a few more wrinkles.

This time, for the first time, I *hoped* for a positive, so why was I just as scared?

7 Positive

There it was. The faint, but undeniable pink line. And another… and another. This was the magical moment I'd dreamed of. I waited for my tears of joy to appear, but I was too shocked to emote. Millions of women struggle with fertility and would do anything to be in my shoes. I knew that.

Wait, I've already done this wrong, I thought. I wished I could rehearse and try again.

Life as I knew it from this moment would be completely different. *POOF* My current life disappeared in an instant, and I didn't get to say goodbye. I wasn't ready to let go of this version of me whom I felt like I'd just met. I thought back to the high of that New York trip. I looked up blankly into the bathroom mirror above the sink where I'd laid out the tests. My eye circles were dark. I looked like shit.

If only I could re-do this and be like the girls on TikTok who filmed themselves reading the positive test. You know the ones. They cover their mouths in shock and jump for joy. A cute piano melody plays softly behind the video. Instead, I stared awkwardly at the sink in silence, not ready to leave the bathroom and face the world with this news. When I'd leave this room, it all would begin like a snowball tumbling down a hill getting bigger and bigger with each second. On one hand, I'd received the best news. It felt like a miracle, but it also suddenly killed the woman I was, and I wasn't supposed to mourn her. I was supposed to dance on her grave, thrilled to be a mom, nothing else, and live happily ever after. I focused on telling Connor and pushed away the feeling I retrospectively recognized as grief.

I was now positive that I was pregnant, but why didn't I *feel* more positive about it?

"When will you be home from the gym? I miss you!" I texted him, trying to act normally.

The more I thought about telling him, I started to get excited. I still felt grief and fear, but finally, there were those butterflies I was supposed to feel earlier too. It was a confusing emotional storm.

"I'm stopping at the store after the gym, so I'll be late."

"Ugh hurry I have a present for you! It's a souvenir from Florida," I lied.

"Ah is it an ornament?"

"Maybe!"

I wished I had the patience to wait and conjure up a more elaborate and memorable announcement. He and the baby deserved the social media worthy video, but I couldn't wait. I had to improvise and keep it simple. I was also still running on fumes from that trip and a long workday on no sleep.

He finally came in the front door with plastic bags full of groceries as the dogs jumped for joy all over the living room, nearly knocking over the Christmas tree. I spotted bell peppers and knew he was about to cook our favorite meal, his low-carb fajita wraps. We hadn't seen each other since I got home from Florida, and I missed him. I was so relieved to be with him and couldn't wait to have him share the load of this huge news I was carrying, quite literally. I settled into a big comforting hug and hoped he wouldn't feel me shaking with nerves.

"Wait just open this first, please," I begged before he poured me a glass of wine I couldn't have.

We always drank the same sweet concord wine together for at-home date nights. On my own, I preferred a dry red like a Chianti or maybe a light white like a Chenin Blanc, but this stuff tasted like Concord grape juice and went down like it too. We loved to be comfy at home and cook and eat together, wine drunk. He assumed this was the agenda again tonight. I'd miss those nights, I thought. We'd never have that again. I'm pregnant now and can't drink for a long time, and when I'm done, we'll have a baby. It won't just be us two anymore. How exciting to think of us as a family of three, but I was gutted to feel the loss of our family of 2. Again, I felt grief that wasn't allowed to be there. Again, I pushed it somewhere deep inside me, that spot in our center where we all store those feelings we aren't ready to feel. I'd have to reschedule the grieving of my own 30-year-old self I'd just started to get to know as well as our relationship as I knew it.

I'd hidden the positive pregnancy tests in a Christmas gift bag. He still had his gym outfit on as he opened them in front of the low cream-colored light of our Christmas tree in our living room. He stared into the gift bag for a few seconds of confusion, probably thinking they were COVID tests at first glance. I watched his face light up when he realized. He smiled, and he was speechless, but his glassy eyes said enough. We both teared up and hugged in silence. There aren't words for a moment like that. I finally felt the bliss I was missing earlier. We suddenly had this precious little secret. I held onto it, stared at my lower belly, and I craved that wine all night long.

8 Now What?

"I'm pregnant so I need to make an appointment for this week, please," I said to the doctor's office, assuming that's what I was supposed to do.

I was whispering in a conference room in our office in between Microsoft Teams calls, peering through the glass, scared that someone might walk by and hear me.

"You can come in after you're about ten weeks, honey" the nurse said after estimating how pregnant I might be based upon my menstrual history.

I learned that they count the pregnancy as beginning on the first day of your last period, which is easier to pinpoint than the actual conception date.

"Okay, and what should I expect at the appointment? I assume we'll take a look at the ultrasound or sonogram or whatever it's called to make sure everything looks okay?" I clutched my pen, prepared to take notes like an eager candidate ready to report for a job interview.

"Ultrasound? There's no ultrasound," she said as if I should know this.

Already, I felt like I didn't deserve this job I was interviewing for. Had I lied on my womanly resume?

"Oh. Well, can I please get one?"

I'd imagined all the ways I'd announce the pregnancy with the printed ultrasound photos I'd seen on social media. A photograph holding them over my belly with Connor's hands wrapped around us, or maybe I'd hide them in something as a surprise for people to open in person. Plus, I wanted to meet this baby inside me and couldn't wait another second longer to not see them. My apps told me the baby was the size of a peppercorn, a sprinkle, and a medley of other tiny edible items to supply my imagination, but I wanted to see the real thing.

"We don't even have the capability to do those here. That would happen at an ultrasound office, and that's only if the doctor decides you need one for some reason. She'd write you a prescription," she said sweetly, but I feel condescended.

This was news to me that women sit in uncertain anticipation like this after taking a pregnancy test for TEN weeks. Then, when we're there, we don't even get to see the baby? How would I know if I'm doing anything right? I rode out the next month and a half in limbo, knowing I was pregnant, but waiting for a medical professional to direct me and confirm all is well in there. I also learned that this isn't necessarily the timeline or routine for everyone. Standards and protocol differ per hospital and/or per state. Some health networks cite unlikely yet possible risks of ultrasound imaging or sonography like the ultrasound waves slightly heating tissue or creating pockets of gas in the fluids. The FDA and WHO recommend limiting exposure to only what is medically necessary. No one was explaining any of this to me. I had to come prepared to calls or appointments throughout the pregnancy with lists of questions I'd pre-researched. I quickly learned women are on their own to educate ourselves on our health and our baby.

My new research project that I felt underqualified to conduct became "How to be pregnant correctly."

9 Maternal Survival

Maternal deaths in the US are more common than in other industrialized countries like Canada, The UK, France, Germany, and many others.

"The US is one of the most dangerous places for women to give birth compared to other countries," article after article shocked me.

My stomach turned as I discovered the US had the highest 'maternal death rate" in the developed world. I thought we had the best healthcare globally. The secret seemed to be that this did not apply to women's healthcare, and this is only common knowledge to women who've been through this process. It's even more dangerous for women of minority groups. Federal data shows that black women's mortality rate in recent years was more than three times the rate for white women and significantly higher than Hispanic and Asian women.

Why isn't anybody talking about this on a larger scale, I wondered. As a woman, how have I never heard of this?

I decided to armor myself with information. I drank from the firehose. I followed every OBGYN, Doula, Labor & Delivery nurse, and mom-influencer I could find. The secrets of pregnancy and motherhood began to unfold. The idyllic vision of pregnancy, birth, postpartum, and motherhood began to crumble to reveal the true experience. Women who'd had babies already began speaking to me differently.

"Pregnancy was the healthiest I've ever been!"

"Being pregnancy is so beautiful!"

"I loved being pregnant!"

These comments I received *before* getting pregnant suddenly turned. It was as though I'd been initiated into a secret society of pregnant women. They could now be honest with me about their experience. When they heard I was pregnant, they could let their mask fall for a moment and breathe like that feeling during the height of COVID when you could finally remove the humid square off your mouth.

"Oh man, you're due in July? Summer heat with pregnancy is brutal. Be careful. I almost died from heatstroke. Make sure you stay indoors with AC," a stranger told me at a graduation party.

"I'm lucky to be alive. I almost died from preeclampsia. Make sure you check your blood pressure and don't let them send you home from the ER if it's high. They'll try to," A friend's wife told me.

"I threw up every day for months and ended up in the ER multiple times. Good luck!"

"Pregnant woman collapses and dies at work," a Daily Mail article read my Snapchat feed. A pregnant teacher died in her classroom, pushed beyond her physical limit. Would she have survived if pregnant women had more rights in the US around work like the rest of the world?

It all appalled me. Women continued to share their near-death experiences with me. However, they assured me that, "All of it goes away as soon as they put that baby on your chest! Don't worry! It's all worth it!"

That moment seemed to buoy women and give them some endurance through pregnancy and labor, so I hoped it would do the same for me.

I immediately bought *What to Expect When You're Expecting,* before realizing I didn't have time to sit and read a book with my work schedule. How do working moms learn all this information, I wondered. I listened to the audiobook every second I could. I hung on every word at 1.5 speed to maximize each minute. 15 minutes while I did my skincare and makeup in the morning. Another 20 minutes on my commute to the office. Another 20 on the way home. I then scrolled relentlessly for two hours before I fell asleep each night through a perfectly curated TikTok algorithm. It actually educated me much faster with tailored information for my age, how many weeks I was, and where I lived. It was efficient, and I found myself grateful for technology like this. I wondered how pre-technology women prepared themselves for such a big life change.

10 Studying

I bought Connor his own parenting book for new dads. While the mom-oriented books were thick and serious like scholarly textbooks, the dad-oriented books were colorful, brief, and silly like they were made for children. This one had a bright yellow cover with a busy cartoon dad on it. Illustrations broke up the dumbed down information about each stage of baby's development. I held Connor accountable every night to read a few pages, as if he was unwilling to do his homework, and the book's childlike artwork began to make sense.

"Have you read your pages tonight?" I asked with an annoyed tone, peeling off one earmuff from his gaming headset. His eyes were glued to his PC. He and his friends played video games like this every night. It was the bane of my existence and that of their wives as well.

"And did you feed the dogs?" I asked, already dreading the answer.

"No, they need to eat," he said, eyes still locked to the screen.

"Great." I rolled my eyes and dragged my exhausted, pregnant, and overworked body to the kitchen to clean messes I didn't make, feed the dogs, and let them outside. I wondered when I'd get to shower. I leaned on the counter watching Punkin snort through his kibble and wondered how a baby would fit into this nightly routine if Connor couldn't realize how much he'd need to step up and change.

"It doesn't become real for the men until the baby is actually here," moms would tell me. "It's all imaginary until then."

Green with envy (and morning sickness)

My educational scrolling evolved into resentful scrolling, jealously following creators who married wealthy men or hit the jackpot with followers. Yeah, I know President Theodore Roosevelt said, "Comparison is the thief of joy," but I wanted to wallow, okay? One particularly beautiful influencer vlogged as she laid in her ornately landscaped in-ground pool, sipping a smoothie that her husband delivered to her on his lunch break. She spent business hours tending to the needs of her pregnant body and mind. Being a budding mom *was* her job. She'd hit the lottery. She minimized stress and focused on nutrition, birthing techniques, meditating, and preparing their home for the little life about to join it. My TikTok algorithm tortured nightly with videos like this of pregnant women who didn't work or weren't chained to a shift, at least. They tended to their bodies' needs and their baby's needs. They seemed so happy. They shopped for baby supplies and clothes at Target in the morning and spent the afternoon organizing and decorating the nursery. I couldn't find any moms who'd be like me. I hope I'm filling some voids like this for you through this book. I stewed in envy and grieved the life I thought my baby and I deserved, the one I wished every mom could choose.

I put my phone down next to me and cried. "I'm so sorry," I said to my baby, wishing I had the time to focus on him or her and our well-being to give us both a good experience. I felt so guilty about the stress, exhaustion, and lack of time I had to properly prepare anything for this baby to arrive.

Later in pregnancy, after I was pregnant enough for the appointments, this envy worsened when my midwives unintentionally reinforced my guilt.

"I recommend about 3 naps per day and more when you feel you need it. Rest is very important for your body right now, so try to give it as much as possible," one midwife advised.

"Frequent small meals throughout the day can help with the nausea you're feeling." But I don't get frequent lunch breaks, I thought.

To combat nausea, a midwife told me the popular medical fix is a mix of Vitamin B6 with Unisom.

"It's basically a sleeping pill, so it will just knock you out and let you nap all day," she said with a smile.

Pregnant women could escape the nausea and puking with all-day naps, like sleeping off a hangover. I'd seen all of those influencers and celebrity moms talk about it.

When I told her I worked fulltime, she offered me a stare of pity. "Oh," she nodded compassionately at my misfortune and adjusted her glasses.

"Just rest when you can then."

11 The Baby Factory

I'd finally made it to that first OB appointment at Magee Women's Hospital, locally referred to as "the baby factory." Hospitals already put most of us into scary-mode, don't they? I knew this one well because my mom had her breast cancer treatment there. I spent much of my childhood in its waiting rooms, head buried in coloring books, innocently unaware of the bleakness that brought me there. The hospital seemed neat to four-year-old me. We'd enter the lobby through the ginormous revolving door. I'd hold my mother's hand and marvel at the bustling lobby and shiny marble floor, the kind princesses must have in their castles. I'd run in my sparkly shoes over to a self-playing piano that greeted patients and families. I thought it was magic or a friendly ghost playing, and my mom didn't dare correct me.

In the doctor's office, they'd take my mom privately to their serious grownup conversations while the nurses distracted me. My favorite nurse was Sarah. I looked forward to seeing her at each appointment like she was a fun and cool big sister. I admired her black box-braids pulled into a long ponytail I could have only otherwise imagined on a mermaid. She taught me how to braid and brush hair, and I'd bring my Barbies for us to practice on. She taught me girly things like hair skills while my mom couldn't and shielded me from the darkness around me. My reverence for and trust in nurses began and persisted with her. I think this was partly why I was afraid to speak my mind in the delivery room.

25 years later, there I was in that big revolving door again. I looked to my right, and there was the self-playing piano. This time my hand wasn't wrapped safely in my mother's. I wished like hell it was and imagined her soft fingertips and freckles. Being at Magee again tore open a wound I didn't realize was so loosely stitched, and I held back tears as I wandered to the correct office.

The doctor took an iPhone-sized screen and pushed around my belly unpleasantly with what looked like a mini ultrasound machine, looked briefly, and said, "Yep, you are pregnant," as if I hadn't gathered that over the last couple of months of hellish symptoms.

"And you've looked into what foods you should be avoiding?"

"Of course!" What if I hadn't? What if I didn't have a TikTok degree in obstetrics to tell me all about listeria in lunch meat or the effects of more than 200mg of daily caffeine? Shouldn't this conversation have happened earlier?

"Any concerns?" she asked.

Not knowing where to start, I blurted out, "I really do not want a C-section."

She scoffed, typing on her computer. "Nobody does, but if we have to, we have to."

It was over in 8 minutes. I'd waited for weeks and missed a whole morning of work for it, and now I had to rush back to the office. It became even more clear that women are in so many ways, on their own to prepare for this giant transformation.

12 First Trimester

I came across a clip of psychologist and author Dr. Julie Smith. She was speaking as a guest on *The Unplanned Podcast* on an episode about the pregnancy and postpartum experience.

"Every cell in your body is pregnant when you're pregnant. It changes everything," she said.

That's the best way to put it. Not a single cell in my body felt the same. I'd been irreversibly changed into something different—I wasn't sure what or who quite yet.

Pregnancy tired

The word "tired" didn't suffice. There's not a word in the English language that accurately describes pregnancy tired. This is especially true for working moms who can't rest the way their body needs. My body and mind were both heavy. One day, my alarm blared to wake me up at 6AM, as it always had. I'd been a "morning person" until pregnancy. I opened my eyes, but I couldn't get them to focus. I blinked, but they moved in slow motion in the dark. I knew I had to get to work by 7:30AM and channeled that anxiety as fuel, hoisting myself to a sitting position on the edge of the bed. My body was begging me to lie back down and let it rest. The dark room spun, and my eyes were blurred. I stood up and fell right back down, backward onto my cotton comforter. I could not get up. I crawled my way to the bathroom and started the day on my knees. You may be wondering…Why not take a sick day? Well, this wasn't just one day. This was my new norm. Excelling at work like

I used to was impossible. I didn't recognize this person I'd become. I fell asleep sitting up at my desk and couldn't find words during meetings. I felt grateful to have a desk job and pitied the women who had physically demanding jobs too where they needed to be on their feet all day. It's not just pitiful. It's dangerous. According to the NIH, studies show that women who are on their feet for much of their workday are more likely for major health risks. In addition to back, feet, and neck pain, many of these women experienced chronic venous insufficiency, preterm birth, and miscarriage.

Mom Brain

One day, I had a first meeting with a potential client, Tracey. She was a stern and cold Operations Director interested in my hiring services.

"Good… morning," I said slowly with a confused expression.

It wasn't an exceptional vocabulary word, "morning," and it should have fallen off my tongue with zero thought. Instead, I had to push and strain to get the word out. I wondered if I was having a stroke.

Tracey looked at me pensively for a moment, and I dove into my sales spiel. I usually had no problem commanding a room in the business world, but this time, every few words got stuck like a clogged pipe from my brain to my mouth.

"I'll send you a… uh…calendar… uh…invite…" I was so embarrassed and figured I had to call out the elephant in the room or risk her thinking I was an airhead and lose her to my competition.

"Okay, I'm so sorry. I'm pregnant and I guess I have mom-brain, please bear with me," I chuckled. "I promise I'm not an idiot."

Her professional expression softened. "Oh, I understand I have a son. I remember what that's like. It's a real thing. The baby eats your brain," she said, leaning into the computer as if she was whispering a secret that she didn't want her coworkers to hear.

We found a moment of connection, and I retrospectively think it's what attracted her to the business partnership, my human honesty, something I hadn't tapped into in my work before. I hung up the meeting and couldn't stop thinking about what she said about my brain.

I'd heard women joke about "mom-brain," but it always sounded like a cutesy forgetfulness. In my Google studies, I learned it's called aphasia, difficulty with language, that varies in severity. Research confirms the brain loses gray matter volume and cortical thickness during pregnancy. An NIH article discussed some research finding lasting changes, especially in the regions that control social cognition. It said, "The results show the volunteers' brains underwent changes on an almost weekly basis during pregnancy."

Other articles, like one from Science.org, said it's beneficial. The brain changes to focus on the woman being a mother, rather than anything else she needed to be before. The study found the most affected areas were the social areas and the hippocampus, associated with memory. The women who'd lost the most volume also showed highest levels of attachment to their infant during testing. What shocked me more was that after two years, the MRI scans on the subjects appeared to show the same loss in gray matter. It was clear that women are forever changed by motherhood. It overtakes them body and soul. How could I be the same employee when neither my mind nor body gave a shit about my work anymore?

Food Aversion

I couldn't eat, and I missed food. The food aversions were particularly stressful because I knew my body needed more nutrients than ever yet couldn't bear the thought of anything but toast. Everything else made me gag, especially water. I went into the office three days a week, which was a schedule I used to love. I had the best of both worlds. Three days of socializing and high-energy and two days of working from home with more focus. I fought nodding off at the wheel on my commute, practiced smiling and strutted my heels into the humming office to play the part. I smelled everyone's perfume and cologne, holding in vomit. I steered clear of the kitchen, holding my breath walking past it. Smelling everyone's lunches sent me over the edge, and I tried to rush my pukes in the shared women's bathroom before other girls came in. No one here had been pregnant before. They wouldn't understand. I couldn't believe women operated like this.

Although joy enveloped me, I noticed a grief that seemed to grow with each new "can't." No more cappuccinos, sushi, deli meat, wine, cocktails, shrooms, weed, soft cheese, Botox… Even my lotions and skincare weren't pregnancy safe. It all had to stop cold turkey. These are all frivolous things and certainly worthy sacrifices for a healthy baby. But they were my favorite things nonetheless, and I watched as every detail of my daily life had changed and become only about baby. The comfort of my own routines was gone. I felt like Marty McFly in the movie

Back to The Future when he sees his hands and notices he's disappearing, ceasing to exist before his own eyes. It wasn't just about missing the crisp and cold first sip of white wine in a thin-stemmed glass, or the drag of a Juul on a rough workday to take the edge off. It was about losing the woman I was. I started to mourn life as I knew it, and it was even heavier having to keep it all a big secret.

Baby Bubble

Connor and I hadn't told anyone, and even though I was sick, it felt special to have our secret love bubble. Every time I left the house, I couldn't wait to get home. Having something that was just between us felt sacred, and I felt closer to him than ever before. We'd lay on the couch at night, and he'd rest his head on my lower-belly. I disconnected from everyone around me, and my instincts were to stay home with Connor, snuggled on the couch. This baby was so pure and innocent, almost holy. I already wanted to protect him or her from the ugliness I knew was out there in the world. I felt delicate and vulnerable. I felt like an utterly different being forced to fit into the world of the person I no longer was.

I couldn't hold this in for much longer. I was bursting with excitement, but the bubble was also lonely. I needed support, a sounding board, anything. I had to lie when people asked me how I was doing or what I was up to.

When someone grieves, they usually don't have to do it alone. Everyone comes over with a casserole and a hug. I needed the casserole treatment, but my casserole friends couldn't understand. I was having a child, but I felt like a child more than ever. I wanted my mom.

13 Denial

My favorite poem is "Do not go gentle into that good night," by Dylan Thomas. It's always ignited a rebelliousness against my own mortality, "Rage, rage against the dying of the light." I recited the line internally and decided I would rage against pregnancy killing the woman I was. I gripped her tightly. Women CAN do it all, and I was going to prove it, I thought.

December was a packed month, a newly pregnant woman's nightmare, but I was determined to remain "fun," so I glued on my lashes and dragged myself through my social obligations. Three family holiday parties, three friends' birthday parties, and two work events. I didn't know it then, but this stage of grief was clearly denial.

I noticed how ingrained alcohol is in our culture. Work happy hours, wine at dinner, open bars at weddings… Would I feel like an outsider everywhere we went now? It wasn't about the alcohol itself. It was lonely when every single other person is in a different mindset, lubricated and freer of inhibitions. I watched everyone grow a bit louder and their words started to slur.

Natalie had another party, this time for her birthday at a speakeasy. The theme was "Diamonds & Fur." We're all about a theme, and we lived to dress up. The excitement I used to feel about getting a new outfit and piecing together an on-theme look was nowhere to be found. Still, I raged on. I squeezed into a fully rhinestoned silver dress with a white fur coat and my favorite satin black pointed-toe heels. I used to love getting ready and remembered the NYC trip, how much fun I had curling my long hair and blending my eyeshadow like a painting. Now, I sat on the floor in between hair sections so I wouldn't pass out. It took me 3 hours to get through my hair and makeup.

I looked in the mirror at the finished product and said to Connor triumphantly, "I fucking did it!"

He didn't hear me over the Saint JHN song he had blasting through the house as he pre-gamed. He was already buzzed, and I felt left out. I couldn't believe I now had to leave the house. Getting ready took all my energy, but it felt like everyone was counting on me to be there. A good friend is someone who shows up, and I'm a good friend, I thought.

This was my first real social outing without alcohol. It was a speakeasy. The whole point of being there is to drink cocktails. It was in a back alley in the hipsterly Lawrenceville area. I could tell Natalie had ahold of the aux because I could hear Future from outside. The door buzzed with the bass as I walked in behind Connor. Quickly, I noticed I was in for a rough ride. It was small and pitch dark with velvet couches on the sides of the room and a small bar in the corner. I yawned, my eyes begging me to lay on those couches and go to sleep. I strategically waited for the bar when no one was there and sighed with relief when I saw a mocktail menu.

"I'll have the *mock* espresso martini, please," I mouthed to the bartender, trying to whisper over the heavy bass of the rap music to keep my cover. From one look at the color, I knew it was basically watered down cold-brew with a bean garnish. It looked legit enough to play it off as the real thing, and that's all that mattered. I just needed a prop. I only drank about half of it, remembering I needed to limit caffeine. By 11PM, Alex and I could not get up off the couches. We were embarrassed and knew we were being lame. Everyone noticed.

"What's wrong with you guys tonight?"

"I feel like everyone hates us," I whispered to Alex.

"That's because they do. We're Debbie Downers. We're ruining the vibe, but I cannot get up. I'll barf," she whispered back.

I smiled, talked to people, awkwardly danced in my seat, and tried my best to perform. I puked in the restroom and held back tears, feeling trapped and torn between the old me and the new one I was becoming. Connor was wasted. I could always tell when he was drunk because he'd rocked back and forth and talked a bit too loudly.

"Love you!" He yelled. I didn't say it back.

I'd imagined, as my partner, he wouldn't drink since I couldn't, and he'd want to leave everywhere early when I was spent. It was evident that his life would go on, while mine flipped upside down. We never talked about these things before because I never imagined I'd feel this way. We imagined I'd feel nothing but maternal joy. I waited for everyone to get drunk enough not to notice me leave, and I Irish-good-byed out the back door.

Two weeks later, we had a friend's birthday party at one of those golf simulator bars. I was dying to tell Carly. I don't keep secrets from her. I got a wine bottle label that said "I can't drink this, but you can" from Amazon to tell my sisters and friends. I felt guilty not telling her and Connor in a more creative way, but I couldn't wait and didn't have the time with work to put together anything more elaborate. It still felt cute and special.

"I have an early Christmas gift that you need to open ASAP. I'm bringing it tonight," I texted Carly.

I was only about 7 weeks pregnant, but I couldn't find pants that fit. Already? I'd never heard of the first trimester bloat. I was painfully inflated with a baby bump, but the baby was only the size of an ice cream sprinkle. I squeezed into my least favorite jeans that were usually too big from the bottom of my drawer. Carly and her boyfriend picked us up to carpool to the party. My heart pounded the whole drive there. She opened it in the parking garage and was so shocked she had to walk around the building and meet us back inside. Her life was about to change too as her best friend became a mom. Would we still have anything in common? We'd entered every stage of womanhood together, but I was leaving her behind for this one. We kept quiet at the party. I sneakily ordered Shirley temples at the bar.

"What are you drinking?"

"Dirty Shirley," I lied.

By the third shot I'd avoided by slipping it to Connor, everyone noticed my sobriety.

"What's wrong?" They all repeated.

"C'mon get drunk and have fun with us! We're going out after this. You're coming!" My friend Megan said.

She tried to buy me another "dirty Shirley" before we just had to tell her too."

One by one, we told our friends, and I watched their eyes light up with excitement.

A few hours in, my fun ran dry. Everything hurt, I was miserable, and trying to hide it, which was more exhausting. I'd given up my resolution to "rage." I was pregnant, I admitted to myself, and I wanted to lay down. Connor didn't understand. He wanted to go out and continue the night the way we usually would.

"Just drink some caffeine," everyone told me.

14 Time to Confess

I read that 30% of all pregnancies end in miscarriage, and 80% of those occur in the first trimester. It was risky telling people before the 12-week finish-line that marks the end of the first trimester, but my therapist told me it would better for people close to me to know so that, if the unthinkable were to happen, I'd have a support system.

"No reason to suffer in secret," she said. I agreed.

I had anxiety every minute, and I begged the baby, "Please stay."

We told our families on Christmas. First up, Connor and I called my dad in the car after Mass. As the phone rang, I felt 16 and like I did something wrong. I wasn't married, living in sin.

"What will my traditional Irish Catholic family think here?" I squeezed my hands over my eyes. "My dad is going to know I've had sex," I worried out loud to Connor before my dad picked up the call.

"You're scared?" Connor laughed and squeezed my hand. "I'm the one who needs to be afraid of him!" The ringing stopped and so did our laughs.

After exchanging Christmas pleasantries, I finally dropped the bomb. The conversation was robotic and uncomfortable for all of us and went as follows:

"Well, we have something big to tell you."

"Okay," my dad said.

"Are you ready?"

"I guess…" he said, knowing something was up.

"We're having a baby!"

"Oh my God… *painful pause* … Okay." I could tell he didn't know what to think and needed to digest. I was his baby. He still saw me as a little kid. I still felt like one. Maybe he was right.

"You're the first person we told today, and we're telling the rest of the family later today."

"Okay… Thank you. Love you guys."

My dad and I had always been emotionally reserved and awkward around big feelings. I wouldn't hear from him for 4 months after this. I assumed he was processing. I don't think most men, especially from his generation, realize what women experience in pregnancy. In his mind, maybe this was just part of my womanly experience. I missed my mom differently than ever before. She was so warm and wore every emotion on her sleeve the way I wish my dad and I could. This would have overjoyed her. I thought I'd experienced grief in all its disguises by now, but this was all so uncharted. I was doing the most adult thing I'd ever done, and yet I feel like a little girl. I felt alone. Even though I was happy, this was the scariest thing I'd ever experienced. I thought I'd feel grown. Instead, I felt childlike, craving my own parents to tell me everything would be okay.

Connor's parents were up next. We weren't nervous to tell them because they'd been begging us for grandkids. We surprised them with glasses that said, "Grandma and Grandpa." They were ecstatic for their first grandchild.

I was emotionally exhausted by the time we got to my sister's house for Christmas dinner. My dad's announcement felt more like a confession and could have been so much better with all of us together.

"It's so going to be a girl!" My sisters, nieces, and aunt tearfully screamed and cheered. It was exciting, but nothing could shake me from missing my mom. I wished I could tell her. She was the only one I wanted to talk to. I furtively wiped my tears on the dark drive home back into the city.

"I feel so much less pressure now that everyone knows, don't you?" Connor leaned back in his seat. "This baby is already so loved."

15 New Year New Me

"Should we just stay home?" Connor asked, exasperated from hearing me complain. He watched me struggle to get myself together, gagging constantly over the toilet in between the steps of my makeup routine. Food repulsed me, yet hunger intensified the nausea. All I could stomach were carbs, my sworn enemy, the cardinal sin I'd abstained from these past few years to lose the life-long weight. I was now too sick to fight it. I'd entered survival mode and felt destined to be fat again.

Last NYE, we rang in 2023 with a VIP section at a club and didn't make it home until 3AM. I thought I'd be hungover until 2024. I felt ten years older this year. Remember how my 30th birthday trip felt like a celebration of my new life? This felt like that girl's funeral. I was usually a positive person, but the hormonal mood swings felt like such a heavy weight on my chest that I couldn't even fake it. My personality was gone. Since the getting-ready ritual always made me feel like myself, I tried my best. I put on makeup and a tight little dress with a zipper held together by prayer. Instead of connecting me to my identity, it felt like a disguise or costume. Even though I looked like myself, a pudgier version, she was gone. It felt like I was living in her shell.

Dinner was at 9PM, which may as well have been 4AM.

"Rage, rage against the dying of the light," I reminded myself.

I gripped my sense of self tightly. If I stayed in on NYE, I'd feel like I was ruining Connor's fun holiday and letting the pregnancy win. I was afraid that, if I stopped going to social events, my friends would slowly forget me.

I drove, of course. I drove everyone everywhere now because they all knew I couldn't drink. It only made sense that I was the "DD," designated driver, at every outing. Little did they know I was so drained and spacey, lest we forget my shrinking brain, that I wondered if I should even be operating a vehicle. I watched everyone drink champagne and eat tuna tartare while I was stuck with water and mint gum to keep me from puking onto the pristine white tablecloth.

I thought pregnancy was supposed to feel amazing. That's what I'd heard all my life, that it's "a beautiful miracle," but I'd never felt so misunderstood, alone, and sick. I couldn't figure out why I wasn't having this magical pregnancy experience. I wish women had been honest with me so that I would have known that all of this was normal. I'd have noticed more of the magic. I imagine that, although I would still be nauseated, the mental and emotional weight would have been lighter. I felt guilty for not loving pregnancy so far.

By midnight everyone was drunk.

"You're being a bitch tonight." Connor was mad at me for my attitude I'd been giving him all night. Remember when I told you earlier that we'd be mad at him soon? This is one of those moments.

I *was* being a huge bitch, on purpose, and I was good at it. He'd taken an ecstasy pill with the rest of the guys at dinner and felt on top of the world. I hated him for it. I felt excluded, like I suddenly had nothing in common with these people and couldn't relate to them all night. If I couldn't do these things, I thought he shouldn't either. I resented him, but I tried to hide my disdain to protect the vibe for everyone.

I was unsuccessful and made passive aggressive jabs at him all night, like, "You're having another drink already?"

I finally got to retreat to my warm safe bed at 1AM. I cried into my pillow, having a New Year's pity party. Despite how much I hated that night, I still imagined the year ahead with my sweet baby. It was an odd feeling knowing something so happy and beautiful would come from feeling so sick and alone. I felt disconnected from the world, only connected to this baby. I dreamt of next year's NYE with my baby, snuggling at home. It would have sounded so lame to the old me that I wouldn't be able to stand it.

"Let's go to the BAR," she'd say.

This was the first night I noticed that, although the woman I'd been was dying, there was another person growing alongside the baby to be born with them. I wasn't ceasing to exist, but I was becoming someone new.

16 Eye of The Storm: Second Trimester

By weeks 13-14, the nausea lifted like heavy smog had passed and the sun came out again. It was like that feeling when your hangover finally goes away in the late afternoon after dying all day on the couch. I could eat again, and nothing could stop me. To celebrate my returned appetite, Connor took me on a dinner date to one of our favorite restaurants, Joseph Tambellini. It's small and cozy in an old house-turned-restaurant with delicious Italian food. It's a perfect winter-date spot, charming and intimate.

"Don't torture her!" Connor jokingly stopped the server as she started to tell us about the wine special that night. A Chianti, my favorite, imported from Italy. I laughed with them both as he pointed to my belly.

"Never mind, it's terrible," she joked back for consolation.

As I delighted in my angel hair pasta that I never would have let myself eat pre-pregnancy, I looked down at my hands. Am I dreaming, I thought. My hands were black.

"What the fuck…" Connor put down his fork and leaned forward. "What's happening?"

Before panicking, I pulled out my phone and headed back to Google, as I'd done for each new surprise symptom the doctors hadn't warned me about. Turns out, this is common. Pregnant women are often low on iron since our bodies give so much to the baby. I was so anemic that their type of silverware turned my hands black where I'd touched it. It happened to my friend Alex too a few weeks

later when her David Yurman bracelet turned her arm
black. Don't you think someone should talk to women
about these things beforehand? How difficult would it be
for even our doctors to say, "Here are some things you may
experience that are totally common or normal." This way,
when we see them, we're not panicked. Let's talk about
some of these things together, you and I, since no one else
will.

Secret Symptoms

The second trimester was mostly blissful. I felt so
much better than I did in the first trimester. One of the
midwives laughed when I told her this and said, "Yes, think
of this as the eye of the storm." However, I continued to be
jarred by some other symptoms of which no one warns us.

- A few of my toenails fell off regularly.
- One of my molars broke.
- Debilitating migraines, which disappeared
  when I supplemented Magnesium at the advice of a
  midwife
- Brown spots all over my hands called
  melasma
- Constipation
- Discharge
- Heartburn and acid reflux
- Nosebleeds
- Leg cramps

Let's keep going because the list goes on, and these are
only the ones *I* personally experienced. Pregnancy can be
different for everyone.

I had the symptoms we do hear about too like cravings.
Those had also kicked in. When I'd heard them in the past,

I'd pictured that feeling of, "Hm I could go for something sweet," after eating a salty meal, or when you hear someone talk about pizza and it just sounds like it would hit the spot. I felt instead like a horror movie character, a zombie mindlessly chasing her need for brains or a vampire fighting the urge to drink blood, never satiated. I wanted carrot cake, and I wanted it fucking now. I often sent Connor on wild goose chases all over the city to find me what I needed. He once found me a carrot cake at 9PM at the drop of a hat and with no hesitation. The problem with cravings were that all other food repulsed me and sent me gagging over the commode. I could only eat that particular thing I was craving. One day it was steak, another day strawberries, another day cereal. I learned that the body will sometimes crave foods that contain whatever nutrients it needs for the baby recipe that day. For example, it may crave strawberries needing folate, or cereal and carbs for iron.

"Have you been craving eating rocks, ice, or any non-edible objects," a midwife casually asked at my next appointment.

She didn't explain, but luckily, I'd stumbled upon the reason in all my Google searches. She was checking for a common disorder pregnant women develop called Pica. I was familiar with it because our dog, Punkin, had it. He ate rocks, toys, and paper towels compulsively. Apparently, it's common in pregnancy due to nutrient deficiencies.

"Just Krispy Kreme donuts," I replied, which to my disordered mind, had always been indeed inedible. Connor once drove an hour to the closest one to get me a whole box.

I was too scared to tell her of my strongest craving of all for fear that I'd truly lost my mind. I craved the smell of fumes, especially from a vacuum cleaner or any machinery. The craving was so strong that I would stay up at night and watch ASMR videos of vacuum cleaners gliding across carpets, wishing I could smell it. I'd stick my face secretly up to air conditioners or any other machinery I could find. I'd drive to random parking garages just to get a whiff. I couldn't satiate it. I know, it's fucking weird, isn't it?

Many women don't speak up about this because they don't know that it's common. They assume they're crazy. This is another instance where this silence is dangerous because cravings like these signal the body's deficiencies.

Again, my TikTok and Google research led me to, yet another obscure yet common pregnancy condition called "desiderosmia." Pregnant women can have strong cravings of fumes like this. It's believed to be caused by iron deficiency, which I was already treating with iron supplements. I remembered the baby was draining me of nutrients. Women literally create babies' bodies from their own, and the world doesn't give them enough credit for it or support to do it.

In the second trimester, I also felt the cuteness of pregnancy. I was excited to see the little belly bump peeking through my sundresses. It made the round ligament pains worth it. The first few kicks were like flutters. I'd gasp and say, "Come feel my belly! There she is! She just moved!" In those months, Claire made her presence known gently. I'd beg her to say hello. I knew she was there in the first trimester, but it sometimes didn't feel real. I couldn't *feel* her yet. By this point, it was now clear she was there, and it opened a huge new horizon of mom-hood.

17 A Girl

We decided that if it's a girl, she'll be Claire and if it's a boy, Marcus. Maybe it was in my head, but everywhere I turned leading up to week 18, I saw the name Claire. A new character on a show I'd been watching, new work encounters, a name tag of a cashier. I imagined a little soul trying to communicate with me from the great beyond. I told her, "I'm listening."

We planned a babymoon trip and wanted to find out the gender on the beach together. We didn't want one of those gender reveal parties with pink or blue smoke spewing out of an explosive, but social media had ingrained in me that this had to be a big moment. We'd have the ultrasound tech write the gender on a piece of paper, give it to Carly, and have her give it to a bakery to bake a blue or pink cake. At the ultrasound office, they had us fill out a form before we started. It was one of those 3D ultrasound places, rather than a doctor's office. I was about 16 weeks now, and I'd waited to see the baby on the screen all this time. The place was cute. It had a big bed with pillows and blankets and a sectional couch. It felt comfortable, not sterile like a hospital room.

I stared at the form. "Do you want us to tell you the gender today? Circle yes or no."

I looked at Connor. I knew we had this whole reveal plan, but I could tell we're both too impatient. His smile told me we were on the same page. I circled "yes." We couldn't keep this secret from ourselves, and I had to know right this second.

The ultrasound tech mentioned her daughter's name is Claire. I hear you, baby, I thought.

The tech kneaded around my belly like a raw sourdough loaf and pushed the baby into the proper position. I wasn't expecting ultrasounds to kind of hurt. I didn't care. I looked longingly at the large flat screen tv where she projected the ultrasound. There was our baby. A real live baby wiggling around in there with fingers and toes. Connor and I hadn't let go of each other's hands, and my whole chest felt warm.

"Are you ready…. You're having a little girl!"

My first shot up like I was fucking Rocky. "Yes!!"

I could feel her moving gently almost like a muscle twitch, but now I could see her and know her name. The tech showed us both the 2D and 3D views. She had her little arms folded behind her head and her feet crossed in front of her like she was lounging by a pool.

"She sure looks comfortable in there," Connor joked, kissing my hand.

Our eyes filled and we stared awestruck at the screen. A little girl. Claire. My daughter. I was immediately in love on a soul level. I would have been happy with a boy too. It wasn't that I needed that particular gender. It was the first real identifier and glimpse at who this little being would be. It was the beginning of her little identity and seemed to wrap it all together. This is the best day of my life, I thought, on the car ride home as I stared at the black and white outline on the prints. Her name is Claire. I'm her mom, and I can't wait to meet her.

18 Splintering

If you feel lonely in your pregnancy or postpartum era, you are not "just hormonal," and you are certainly not alone. In fact, there are many studies about it. I read an article from the National Library of Medicine called "Loneliness in pregnant and postpartum people and parents of children aged 5 years or younger: a scoping review."

These medical studies referenced in the article found that 82% of new parents (yes, dads too) always or often felt lonely. These scientists found that breastfeeding mothers felt the most isolated. It said that mothers felt those around them "lacked empathy for the difficulties."

Points like these are why I'm talking to you about all this. Our partners, friends, and employers lack that "empathy for the difficulties," I think, not because they're heartless, but because they just don't *know*. How can they know when women keep all these secrets? So, let's keep chatting, shall we?

Tinx coined a term called "The Splinter Era," for friend groups. It refers to the chasm between once closely bonded women in their thirties and early twenties. Each friend splinters in different directions as they each embark on life's milestones like moving in with a partner in the suburbs instead of with roommates in the city, becoming single when the other friends are getting married, or the sharpest splinter of all, getting pregnant.

I hadn't experienced a splinter before pregnancy. For the first time in my life, I felt disconnected from my girlfriends who'd previously been my lifeline. Without my mom, they'd become my source of nurturing comfort and support that women effortlessly embody. Now, they didn't understand me, they couldn't. I was so grateful to have Alex, and I couldn't believe we were pregnant at the same time. She was due one day after me, and we couldn't have planned this if we tried. It was fun to send each other nursery ideas and follow the sizes of our babies each week with our apps, but it was also an emotional support I didn't know I'd need. In my opinion, every pregnant woman needs at least one pregnant buddy. Alex was mine.

Aside from my buddy, by my second trimester, I felt like a complete outsider in my friend groups. I'd sit at the lunch table at work and have nothing to add to the conversations and missed inside jokes about what happened at the bars at 2AM that past weekend, or what guy they hooked up with, or what plans they had this weekend. I clung to Alex, who I knew would be the only one who gave a shit that Claire was now the size of a clementine or a macaron that week.

One of my favorite things to do with my girlfriends was go to dinner and drinks in the city at whatever new trendy spot we'd discovered with strong cocktails, truffle fries, and good music. I loved restaurants. I had a huge list on my phone with all the restaurants, cafes, wine bars, and speakeasies in the Pittsburgh area, and I'd check them off with an emoji one by one after visiting. When people asked what my hobbies were, I dared to say going to restaurants, and there was nothing I loved more than a girls' night. When Barcelona Wine Bar opened a location in Pittsburgh, I was so excited to go. It had been on the list in bold font for weeks. I didn't care that I couldn't drink the wine because I was in it for the overall experience and the yummy food. I was sure they'd have a mocktail anyway. I had been sending the 'coming soon" Instagram posts to my friends for weeks.

"Is anyone free to grab dinner and drinks at Barcelona next weekend? It's finally open!"

Strangely, I didn't get a response. The group chat usually would fire back in seconds, and I was expecting at least a few "fuck yeah" replies. Maybe no one saw my message or was busy at work, I thought.

Carly finally came to my desk at work the next morning. I could tell as she sighed and looked out the window behind me that she had bad news.

"So… no one knew what to say in the chat yesterday because they'd all already made plans to go to Barcelona. We already have reservations."

She continued with a phrase pregnant women hear a lot, "We didn't think you'd want to go."

I was hurt and tried not to show it in my face. "Awkward. Who's all going?"

"I mean, everybody but you and Alex, but I asked and they're going to see if we can add two people to the reservation!"

I went, unsure how to say no, but I felt unwanted. Pregnancy continued to break my adult confidence. I could have never imagined the ways becoming a mom would suddenly uproot me from my social circles. Pregnancy is a major undertaking during which moms need their friends the most, and yet, it's when they feel most separated from them. Connecting with other moms is crucial for mental and emotional stability. Finding new ways to connect with your friends also helps. You simply won't be the friend who can be up all night at the bars drinking with them anymore, but you can be the friend who goes for a walk, grabs coffee, or watches a movie. I hope that you can find that friendship

and understanding in me here. I hope also that, now that
you'll see this divide coming, you and your friends can
prepare for it and work your new circumstances into your
social planning.

Birth Class Connections

I'd read wordy medical articles, Reddit pages, blogs,
and baby books and watched hours of TikToks from
OBGYNs, midwives, doulas, L&D nurses, and mothers
about birth; how to prepare for it, how to do it, what it
would feel like, how to advocate for myself, what to avoid,
and all the old wives' tales about it. I felt like I knew
everything under the sun for someone without actual
medical education or knowledge. I even scheduled a birth
class for Connor and me to attend at the hospital, more so
for him, since I knew he hadn't educated himself the way I
had.

After we paid $80, Connor and I waddled into Magee
Hospital. He carried my giant pink pregnancy ball that
seemed to match my giant pregnant belly. It was after work
on a Friday night, and we were both exhausted from our
long workdays. We had a 3-hour class that night, followed
by an 8-hour class the following Saturday morning. This
was their "weekend intensive class," probably targeted for
working moms' schedules. The other class option was a
much gentler 5-day course, where each class was only 1
hour each morning. I once again envied stay-at-home-
moms who had the flexibility of schedule like that.

I looked around the room and immediately felt
connected and seen for the first time in a way my friends
couldn't provide. I noticed a blonde woman walking in late,
limping as fast as she could. Another, barely fitting on her

chair, panted and hurried her husband as he took out a bulk-sized container of Tums to ease her heartburn. Another mom had something called "HG," or Hyperemesis Gravidarum, where she vomits incessantly all the way through pregnancy. It can be fatal, and some women need to have a port of Zofran just to keep down enough nutrients to survive. I thought about how society uses the cutesy name of "morning sickness," when these conditions can become so serious. I wondered also how I'd be able to pay our bills if I'd gotten it and couldn't work. She sat next to a trash can, pale-faced, ready to puke at any moment. I watched as we all occasionally took deep breaths, gasping for air every minute or so. Every woman in this room was just as swollen, tired, anxious, and stressed about birth as I was. I loved it. They all knew exactly how I felt. I think Connor regarded the dads in the room similarly. They all had suddenly lost the partner they knew, who'd been replaced by someone overworked, overtired, nauseated, hormonal, and twice the size as their former.

The instructor broke us into groups for an ice breaker.

"We'll all need to get comfortable around each other. We're about to start talking about our mucus plugs and bowel movements," she said as the crowd politely chuckled.

"Let's each think of the best thing we didn't expect and the worst thing we didn't expect from pregnancy. Write these down on your notepads, and we'll share with our small groups."

Connor and I gathered in our group, a circle of 4 couples.

The first mom, the blonde who walked in late, went first.

"Mine might be different from everyone's. The best part has been getting to feel the baby move inside me," she said looking down at her belly. "It's like our special bond that no one else can feel."

We all nodded touching our own bellies.

"The worst part wasn't even the physical stuff. It was the isolation," she continued.

The rest of us looked down at our notebooks and nodded.

"My friends and family didn't react the way I thought they would, and I've felt very alone and misunderstood," she elaborated.

"I actually wrote the exact same things," the next mom said. "All my friends went to college together, and then, we worked together. I'm no longer able to work because childcare is more expensive than my annual salary. I've had to leave that whole entire life behind," she wiped a tear from her freckled swollen face. "I don't see them much anymore, and when I do, we have nothing in common like we did before."

I prayed I wouldn't be up next because I was holding back tears. I assumed we'd commiserate about acid reflux. Instead, this was the first time the isolation I'd felt was validated and not written off as me being hormonal or dramatic or negative. This was the first conversation I'd been a part of with a tone of understanding and solidarity. It was the first time I wasn't reminded to, "Just be grateful for your healthy baby!" I came there for breathing exercises to help me through labor pains but got so much more—moral support.

Baby Shower

Remember that scene in *Sex & The City* where the girls go to their old friend's baby shower in the suburbs? The episode depicts the non-mothering main characters as a different species than the mommies, to whom they could no longer relate. They used to know these women well, yet they had absolutely nothing in common anymore. They dressed differently and had different hobbies and interests. They moved out of the city and into the suburbs, where Connor and I were headed too. The city girls attended but felt wildly out of place in their dark leather trench coats and crop-tops, contrasting the pastel cardigans and pearls on the moms. The characters saw motherhood as a shattering new identity, and the baby shower prompted reflection. A baby shower or a wedding can polarize any friend group of women because it offers a mirror for their own obligatory social speed.

In the episode, Carrie wrote, "As I watched Laney tear open a terry cloth baby bib with the same enthusiasm she once reserved for tearing off rock stars' pants… I couldn't help but wonder… Was I next?"

Approaching my own baby shower, I worried about the same rift within my own circles.

"With you and Alex pregnant, I feel so behind," Carly told me.

I knew my friends still loved me, and I knew they were trying to navigate this splintering as best they could too. It was hard for all of us. They were grieving the friend who had the time and energy to talk on the phone for hours, or the coworker who would brighten a hard day with a spontaneous martini happy hour. They missed the old me too. They didn't know what I was feeling or thinking, because, as I keep mentioning to you, women keep it all a secret. New moms need the friends who say, "I can't understand what you're feeling, but I'm here."

They all showed up to my baby shower enthusiastically dressed in pink with arms full of gifts for my daughter. I started to feel the support I'd needed, not from the gifts, but their presence and excitement. The love rippled months later when I'd read Claire a book they brought or wrap her in the hooded towel they'd given us. Through these shower gifts, I felt them in the room with me on nights when bedtime didn't go as planned or I felt hopeless.

Nesting

The day after the shower, my SUV was completely packed full like Tetris. Pretty pink satin and pastel fabrics spilled out all over the house like it was one big Vittorio Reggianini painting. It was a gorgeous mess. Connor and I were completely overwhelmed. Carly and our other high school friend, Leah, came over to help me "nest." It's another third-trimester pregnancy symptom. Women feel an intense urge and compulsion to clean and prepare the home for a baby. When I needed to be organizing work calls, my instincts instead told me to scrub baseboards or move furniture. It would hit me sometimes at 3AM that we just *had* to rearrange our dining room right then and there.

"Let's do a nesting party!" Leah told me.

The girls and I walked up the stairs to my bedroom. Connor and I had moved things around so that one section of the room was still ours, and an alcove off the to the side with a window would be Claire's. It would be her little nursery until we could move into a new house with more bedrooms.

The last time the three of us girls were all together in this exact room was probably in 2011. The room had dark pink walls then, and we had feathers in our hair and too much bronzer on our cheeks, probably preparing to sneak out and drink Four Lokos in someone's backyard. One time, Leah and I were doing our makeup there on the floor. I was trying to apply her liquid black eye liner, but we couldn't stop laughing enough to focus. I think we were high. Twelve years later, there she was in the same spot assembling my unborn baby's diaper caddy, while Carly organized her clothes by age. My eyes filled admiring the scene.

Despite this inevitable splintering of friend groups in our thirties, some friends show up for you, no matter the ebbs in flows and what you have or don't have in common. I realized how important these friends are. Even when they can't understand what the other is going through, they show up in their own way. Try to be honest with your friends about what you're feeling and what you need. They can't read minds. Cherish those who tackle it all alongside you. True support comes from those who don't just show for celebrations but rage against life's splinterings.

19 Babymoon

In February, the hot sun was beating on my skin, and for a Pittsburgher this time of year, it was sensational. It was freezing and gloomy back home, but I was baking in the pool at The Savoy Hotel in Miami Beach. I closed my eyes and pretended for a moment that I was that influencer I used to watch on TikTok, unemployed and pregnant, floating in her backyard while her husband served her. I looked at my belly peeking like a little dome above the water's surface. I hadn't needed to wear a one-piece suit like this in years. I felt like I was 12 again watching girls around the rest of the pool. They'd prance around in their bikinis while boys flirted with them and teased me for being fat. I touched my little belly bump to make it as obvious as possible that I was pregnant this time. I slipped on my Dior sunglasses I'd bought myself as a present after surviving the first trimester. They were somehow a gift from 30-year old me to that 12-year-old me. "If we're going to be fat, we're going to chic about it, dammit," I told her. I stirred my melting watermelon smoothie wishing like hell it was a pina colada. The weightlessness relieved my lower back pain, and I never wanted to touch land again. Connor was on his 4th cocktail, laying on a pink lounge chair in the sun and discretely hitting his weed pen.

I could see my phone blowing up on the lounge chair from the water. My clients and colleagues knew I was out-of-office, but I was the only one who controlled my book of business, and my business partnerships were mine alone. It was the perfect job for an anxious control freak like me. I was wrapping up my second trimester, and in just a couple of months, I'd have to completely let go. It was getting easier than I thought it would. I'd always been a martyr at work, but I'd started to disengage. Nothing mattered to me anymore the way this baby girl did. I'd tied my sense of survival and self-worth to my work performance, but she was slowly freeing me from these mental patterns, rewiring me. I imagined staying there at the beach, changing my name, and just never going back to it all. I laughed to myself because last April I was scantily clad in Miami with my girlfriends skinny dipping in our Airbnb pool or stumbling home from LIV at 4am. There I was less than a year later, sober, 25 pounds heavier in a one-piece, unable to walk properly because the baby had pinched a nerve in my back, a common symptom after the second trimester. Alex and I shared the same limp for a few weeks.

I leaned on my arms on the edge of the pool and kicked my legs behind me, enjoying the weightless movement. I wondered if this is how Claire felt in her amniotic sac. I hoped she was just as comfy and enjoying this smoothie as much as I was. I watched all the un-pregnant people freely enjoying their vacations around the pool-bar and wondered what this trip would be like if I weren't pregnant. Connor and I would be drunk on the beach together. We'd stare at the sunset on shrooms and marvel at the teal and pink colors in the sky and ocean. We'd explore the bars, have fun sex, and go to bed late. I was sad that we never got to have a trip, just the two of us, before we became parents. We'd only traveled in groups for weddings or work trips, using the preciously limited days of PTO. We'd never made the time for the two of us, and soon, it would never be only the two of us again.

Connor had never been to Miami. Instead of the classic club-filled wild Miami itinerary, we ate early dinners, grabbed snacks from CVS and settled into bed by 9PM, the latest I could fathom. Our mornings were nice. I limped alongside him to the local coffee shops for a small latte with half decaf, and we enjoyed the calm beach while the rest of the city was still hungover in bed or still at the club.

"I finally feel like a real pregnant person," I told him, cupping my belly as people smiled at us on the beach.

"I'm jealous that you get to feel her!" He said this a lot. I think he felt left out of the experience sometimes and lonely in his own transition into his new identity of dad.

"I'm sorry I can't go out and be more fun," I said.

"What do you mean? I'm having the best time with you girls," he said, squeezing my hand. I could tell he meant it, and I noticed he wasn't itching to go out and live the lifestyle of our 20s like I worried he would.

We talked to Claire and told her all about our trip, and how we'd come back with her. I always made a wish at the beach and threw seashells into the ocean. The vastness of the sea reminded me of a giant well where I could cast my wishes like messages in bottles for the universe to guide ashore. I started as a kid and never outgrew it. I used to wish for money or to be skinny, shallow worldly desires. This wish weighed on my chest. My heart itself felt bigger than ever and my core felt physically deeper. I'd gathered up a bunch of tiny white shells throughout the day. I tossed them, holding my growing belly, and wished for a strong life-long close relationship with my daughter. I'd never wanted anything more. I imagined what my current relationship could have been with my mother if she were still alive. We'd talk on the phone, I'd visit with her often, and we'd go out to eat like we did when I was a kid. I wanted that for Claire and me. I imagined us as mother and daughter through each season of her life. I couldn't wait to know her.

20 The Mirror

"Aw, Katie those look so painful," Connor came toward the bathroom door looking down at the giant globe hanging off my torso.

"Get out!" I slammed the door shut. I was humiliated that he saw me wallowing in the mirror. I had the perfect baby belly throughout my entire pregnancy. I used every serum, oil, cream, and butter, determined to preserve my skin from stretch marks.

"You should know, stretch marks are really just genetic," the midwives warned me.

I thought I'd escape it. I'd made it this far, and thought I was safe… Until 37 weeks. I felt my flesh tear under the skin with every bend or twist. The worst was going to the bathroom and having to struggle to circumvent the belly to wipe. That day, while trying to wipe my ass, already humiliated, I felt the skin on my left side split. The mirror confirmed I was permanently changed. Thick, jagged vertical ribbons of maroon and purple painted my entire lower belly and down through lady bits. The canvas itself was already disturbing. I didn't recognize my shape. My identity had been centered around the goal of being skinny my entire life. Now, skinny wasn't achievable. I was a blimp. Sometimes, it was freeing like I could finally give up the chase, but mostly, it just felt like accepting defeat. My body didn't belong to me anymore.

"Let me in. I don't care. Let me see," Connor said softly.

I opened the door reluctantly peeking one eye at him. "I'll never be the same," I said through sobs.

"It looks like you were attacked by a lion like big claw scratches. Wow," he said. He has a way with words, doesn't he?

"Shut up, Connor!" I slammed the door again afraid he'd never be attracted to me. No one likes a permanently stained blouse or an upholstered couch with torn cushions, damaged goods. He opened the door slowly.

"It's okay. I love you, so what else matters?" He hugged me from behind with his hands on my belly. His touch stung across my skin that was bursting at every cell, but I let him hold me.

The mirror showed me a stranger. I'd gained 65 pounds in pregnancy and saw numbers on the scale that I never dreamed I'd allow myself to reach. I didn't even recognize my own face. It was just as puffy as the rest of my body. I had what women refer to as "pregnancy nose." I read that it's a hormonal phenomenon in pregnancy that can drastically change a woman's face. Estrogen dilates the blood vessels, causing swelling. It appears thicker, wider, and more bulbous. For some women, it can even cause pregnancy rhinitis. The Ohio University Health page described rhinitis as congestion, sneezing, runny nose and post-nasal drip. It all persists through pregnancy like one long cold.

"It will all be over when the baby comes out," everyone told me.

Stretch marks, though, were permanent. They could fade in color, but they'd always be there. Pregnancy had forever marked me like branded cattle. It was the last kiss of death to the woman I used to be and confirmation that I'd never fully get her back. I imagined all my friends in their bikinis this Summer. Most of them were on Ozempic and at their absolute fittest. I never wanted to leave the house again.

Women generally already endure heavy cultural pressure to look perfect. In pregnancy, our control over our ability to achieve these standards disappears. As a result, so does our confidence. I wished I'd known.

21 Losing Steam

As the third trimester countdown waned, I was physically as shambled as my mental state. I warned new clients at the start of meetings that I was pregnant and would inevitably lose my breath during our call. I used to feel confident and knowledgeable in front of these fancy directors and executives. I could see their pity as I gasped for air. I was weak.

"Do they take me seriously knowing I'll be going on maternity leave soon? Wouldn't they rather have a childless 25-year-old who could work until 8pm to get the job done the way I used to do?" My mind raced with insecurity.

"You're still pregnant?"

"Yeah...."

"Wow you're so strong for still working!"

This conversation played out once every 30min, every day, for about three months. The exchange irritated me. Did they think I wanted to be even sitting upright let alone working a 10-hour day? I'm here because I *have* to be, I wanted to say. Don't put salt in the wound every time you see me.

"When do you go on maternity leave?" The repetitive parley continued.

"When I got into labor."

"Haha no, really. When?"

"Really, when my water breaks."

"...What?!?"

"Yeah... That's how it works in the US. Anyway, about this invoice..."

Counting Kicks

I couldn't focus during any of these conversations anyway because my strict homework from the hospital in the last trimester was counting kicks. Pregnant women are expected to count how many kicks they feel per minute and log any changes in frequency. Decreased movement can signal that something is wrong. There are apps to help women keep up with this all day, reminding them so they don't miss a beat. Every time we wouldn't feel our babies very much for a moment, Alex and I would text each other anxiously. We'd pretend to work and keep afloat professionally, but our minds and bodies were focused inward.

"This is such a stressful time," she said.

Tracking fetal movement and catching any of these changes early can save the baby's life. Missing it due to distractions, including work-related, can have immense cost. In many other countries, women can stop working before this point to focus on their and their baby's well-being. How can we expect working moms to focus while getting through the work day? I shuddered wondering if this setup had contributed to the unique American maternal and infant death rates.

It was clear that people didn't realize that the US doesn't have legislation protecting mothers like the rest of the world. Especially with men, it never crossed their minds that maybe we should treat pregnant women differently in the workplace until they saw one in real life. They looked at me pitifully shocked.

"I've never really seen a woman this pregnant working before. I always kind of assumed you'd be out of here by now," a peer told me. "You have me thinking about my wife and what we'll do when we start a family."

It's obvious and bipartisan that women and babies deserve more, isn't it? Women need to stop hiding their experience so that people realize the enormity… before they see a pregnant woman suffering through a long shift, or trying to pump in her car, or being rushed to the ER in an ambulance because she had to return to work before fully healing. This is the real story of working moms today.

Rushing it

Everyone around me seemed impatient. I wanted to wear a t-shirt or walk around holding a sign that said, "Yes I am still pregnant, I'm overdue, no I don't know when my water will break, yes I am still working until that happens, and yes, that is how maternity leave works in the US if we get any at all."

It felt like I was letting everyone down without an answer, inconveniencing teams and clients by not having an exactly predicted time of birth. I couldn't schedule or plan anything with any guarantee that I'd be there.

I listened to coworkers in my same role in Canada and Europe discuss their maternity leaves being 12-18+ months, plus paternity leave dads could use afterward, plus weeks they'd have off while pregnant. I remembered their free healthcare. It all infuriated me. Why did America seem to hate pregnant women? I thought.

My whole body hurt, and I hadn't slept more than 30min at a time in months. It was tough to breathe and speak. My swollen legs and feet looked like they'd burst open with each step. I needed to pee every 15-30 minutes, but I didn't have time to do that during the workday, so I let myself get dehydrated. I had to work through these symptoms with the same expectations as I had before. Non-pregnant me could run laps around this version of myself. How could American society expect me to prepare my body for birth and my home for a baby? After all, birth is life threatening to both of us, especially in the US with high death rates. I was scared, and I was mad. It was unfair to Claire, to me, and to all pregnant women. My heart ached for a better experience for all of us. It still does.

Those cute, gentle flutters I mentioned in the second trimester had now turned into punches, kneading, and pulls that took my breath away. For some time, her foot was stuck under the left side of my rib cage. Remembering babies can break their mothers' ribs in the womb, I breathed and moved carefully. I had carpel tunnel in my wrists that hurt so much it woke me up throughout the night, another common experience from swelling no one warned me about. Swelling turned out to be far more than the cosmetic inconvenience I'd always imagined it to be. One day, I lost complete strength and mobility in my arms. I woke up unable to move them like long heavy noodles attached to my shoulders as dead weight. I shimmied, nearly limbless, to my phone and called the midwives and OB nurses like I'd done a hundred times with each new surprise.

"That's normal," a phrase I'd heard from them so many times. "It's the swelling. Did you eat a lot of sodium yesterday?" I remembered I ate a sleeve of Ritz crackers when I didn't have time to stop for lunch.

"Your blood pressure sounds normal. Just call back if that changes," the nurse said.

I finished my workday as best I could without much access to my arms and thought again about the litany of symptoms women never share with one another out of shame or embarrassment or a need to prove that "we can have it all" or that we can perform at the same level as our non-pregnant peers and competitors. I was afraid to admit how I really felt to anybody. I couldn't tell my family and friends. I'd either scare them or be seen as ungrateful for my healthy baby. I *was* grateful. I wouldn't confess in the professional space either because I knew I couldn't perform well anymore. I didn't want to be passed up for opportunities or prevent people from wanting to partner with me. I'd already been passed up for a promotion due to the timing of my maternity leave. A spot was opening in management in the Fall, but I'd be gone.

"I want you to know that I thought of you first, but given the circumstances, it just wouldn't work," my director told me. He was right.

I was physically and emotionally spent, but I grounded myself with gratitude that my baby was healthy. It would all be worth it to meet her.

Parental Leave Covers

Getting someone to cover for me on maternity leave was awkward. I was lucky enough to work for a "progressive" company that offered minor financial incentives for those taking on a mom's book of business while she was out. How could I ask someone to take on the

60 hours of demanding work I handle weekly for 12 weeks in my absence on top of their own? It's not truly possible.

"I'd love to help you, but I just don't have time to do my job and yours," a peer told me.

In a fast-moving industry and relationship-based sales role, I knew my work would suffer in my absence, but I'd hoped my team could keep it afloat. Some companies hire a temporary contractor to fill the gap for non-sales related roles. In most cases, I've noticed women feel guilty getting pregnant for this reason. They know someone will need to pick up their slack. I remember going to dinner once with a group of girlfriends from college, and some of them were pregnant. I've intentionally left their names out for reasons that are about to be obvious.

"How have you been doing with hiding it at work?" a friend leaned over our Thai food to ask another.

"I'm showing too much, so I'll have to tell them soon, but I think I made it far enough to where they can't find a reason to fire me!" She replied like this was a victory, and the other girls nodded.

"But that's illegal… They can't fire you for getting pregnant, right?" I asked.

The table of women looked at me, shocked at my naivety.

"Obviously, it's never the reason on paper," one explained. "At our company, they typically watch pregnant girls like a hawk. They wait for them to fuck up or come up with some reason to let them go as early as possible so they don't have to deal with it. They just replace them."

"It's the same at my company," another agreed.

"Me too," said another.

I hated that I wasn't surprised. I'd coached and corrected a few of my own clients against wanting to

replace pregnant employees in the past. I felt grateful that I
never feared this at my own company, but it enraged me
that this is the general climate for new moms in the
workforce. I had to make room for a new person to live in
my body, in our home, and now in my professional world
too. It all felt so daunting.

Couvade Syndrome

As I'd suspected I would, I watched Connor's life go
on as nothing was different these last several months. He
joked that he thought he might have Couvade Syndrome.
The National Institutes of Health said it's a condition in
which men experience some pregnancy symptoms
alongside their partner such as weight gain or headaches.

He'd say, "I really need an ice cream tonight. Must be
because we're pregnant!"

We'd laugh, but this was secretly much deeper for me.
Aside from a bit of weight gain, his body remained the
same. His career trajectory, the same. His social groups, his
hobbies, his vices, were the same. He didn't experience the
gravity of pregnancy or soon to be parenthood that I did.
He didn't feel any of the urgency or panic. I felt the weight
of it for all three of us. He played video games and went
out with our friends to bars and football games while I
painted multiple rooms in our house, cried in the mirror,
writhed in pain, begged colleagues to take my workload
while I was on maternity leave. It wasn't his fault that he
was a man, but it was becoming harder not to resent him.
This is so common for couples, and I wished that we were
more prepared.

Prepping

When I wasn't at work, I researched what comes next in pregnancy, what I should do, eat, drink, and what not to do, eat or drink, and, by this point, I started to prepare for the biggest event of it all, birth. By the time I was full-term, I had it all planned. I hadn't let myself lean back in a chair in months because I read that sitting forward with my pelvis perfectly under me would keep the baby in the right position for birth, head-down. I ate 6 dates a day, drank 2-4 cups of red raspberry leaf tea and pineapple juice, took primrose oil both orally and vaginally (yes I shoved it up there), massaged my perineum with a wand, curb-walked, squatted, and bounced on my pink birth ball.

"I hope those work for you," one of the midwives told me smiling. "Many women say they do, but it's not well studied. The only thing that is backed by actual science is to have sex." Connor raised his eyebrows and smirked at me as we listened.

"The trick is though that both of you have to have an O," she said. "That's what produces the Oxytocin and sends the body into labor."

I almost laughed at her. These days, I had sex with Connor as often as I could bear, but I could physically only lay on my side in a fetal position (no pun intended).

Women who are stressed, have trouble going into labor naturally. Working women in their third trimester are probably, I'd argue, the most stressed people out there. Stress hormones, known as catecholamines, delay and disrupt labor. The NIH has multiple medical articles about it. In the wild, it would ensure that we wouldn't go into labor while being chased by a predator. Unfortunately, working women know that our adrenal system can't tell the difference between being hunted by a tiger or a looming deadline. This is also believed to be the reason women most often go into labor at nighttime when Cortisol levels decrease.

I saw what I was up against, and that stressed me out *more*. It didn't matter if a method was science-based or an old wives' tale. I tried it all. I needed to hurry up and go into labor so I could finally tell everyone at work the plan. I'd do it naturally with just the epidural as intervention, and vaginally was my only option.

My strict regimen surpassed past my due date, and I started to consider that interventions might be in my near future.

22 Birth Plan

"Print out your birth plan and give it to the staff when you arrive at the hospital or they will not follow it!" Doulas, nurses, and burned moms passionately warned me in the underbelly of mom-TikTok where women shared their secrets.

"Protect yourself legally if they push any procedures on you without your consent. Have someone in the room to fight for you like a doula," they said emphatically.

"Do you have your birth plan laid out? Have you had an attorney look at it?" Friends of mine who are nurses grilled me.

"Well, I want to survive, I want my baby to survive, and I do not want a C-section," I responded at first, thinking that would suffice, but I learned how important it seemed to have something more detailed.

Educated women take these very seriously because informed consent is often ignored in the delivery room. This much was clear in these discussions. I couldn't believe it. I thought that everyone wanted what's best for the mom and baby, so why is there so much trauma in the delivery room. Traumatized moms detailed receiving procedures like an episiotomy after saying no when it wasn't medically necessary. The doctors would cut their vagina with scissors to pull the baby out faster as the mother screamed "no" in agony. A friend of mine had a family member in the middle of a lawsuit against a local hospital network after doctors practiced the vacuum on her baby's head during a C-section. Vacuums are used in vaginal births, but the doctor let the medical students practice it anyway while the mom laid open on the table, unaware. Her baby's head was permanently disfigured. I shuddered at each story, but I refused to turn a blind eye. I knew I was giving myself anxiety about birth and that not every medical professional was out to get me, but I wanted to know every possible outcome. I wasn't afraid of the individual staff members, but rather the overall system that organized it all, and I couldn't believe I needed to formulate some sort of protection from it on paper.

What's in a birth plan?

Common birth plans include safer birthing positions, delayed cord clamping, skin to skin contact, and delayed bathing, just to name a few. Standard practice for delivery and post-delivery differ per hospital, which is why birth plans are considered crucial in the mom community. I was shocked to learn there wasn't one true modern and accurate protocol for every little thing. It's up to women to research their own hospital's guidelines and standard operating procedures to compare with others, which aren't clearly outlined for the public on their websites. For example, birthing position differs. Prior to the 18th century, most women gave birth upright or on birthing stools, using gravity and the body's natural ejection through contractions. In the 1700's, French King Louis XIV enjoyed watching women give birth. It was rumored he had a "kink" for it. Lying down gave him the best view, and this created the long-lasting medical norm in Western society. Today, it also offers the doctors the most convenient access and visibility. However, studies show that more upright positions are safer, less painful, and more efficient for both the mother and the baby. I read a PBS article discussing it as, "common sense." Lying on the back during pregnancy is discouraged because it compresses the major blood vessel to the uterus (the aorta), yet hospitals lay women down like this for birth, impeding blood flow to the uterine muscle.

"Not compressing the aorta translates to optimal blood flow... which results in maximally useful contraction forces," the article detailed.

Giving birth lying on the back is also the most painful position. I read dozens of articles and studies and watched videos from birth coaches and doulas. X-Rays show the pelvis widens and labor shortens when squatting or staying on all-fours.

"The evidence largely suggests that lying on your back during birth prolongs labor, and slows contractions, yet the majority of women in the US give birth in this position," I read.

Another hospital norm that seemed to defy medical evidence is immediate cord clamping and cutting. It's usually done in the US as soon as the baby is out. Science tells us instead that delaying it for 1-5 minutes or until it stops pulsing increases blood flow to the baby with benefits including improved oxygen circulation to organs. Studies have shown that it increases their blood volume and iron stores, reducing the risk of anemia in the first 6 months of life, according to the World Health Organization.

These weren't niche studies only pertaining to crunchy moms, these were globally recognized findings, yet American birth seemed outdated.

23 C-Sections

The one thing I knew about C-sections was that I didn't want one, but since it was becoming so common, I figured I ought to educate myself further. I hated what I found. In the US, about a third or more of women end up on the operating table for a c-section. CDC data from 2022 showed that the states with the highest probability are in the South; Louisiana, Mississippi, Georgia, and Florida with ranges from 35.12%-38.5% of all recorded births being cesarean. I was in Pennsylvania with an average of 28.36-31.1%.

"More than a third, damn," I thought with a pit in my stomach, daydreaming nightmarish visions of myself cut wide open on the table feeling every pull and cut.

These rates were significantly higher than the World Health Organization's recommended rate of 10-15%. The WHO even provides recommendations for hospitals to avoid "unnecessary C-sections." Their website recommendations include "requiring a second medical opinion for a caesarean section decision in settings where this is possible," and even "financial strategies to equalize the fees charged for a vaginal birth and a caesarean birth."

I rolled my eyes reading the financial points, remembering the corporate nature of our healthcare system I once trusted. The overall sentiment seemed to be that hospitals want you in and out as quickly and efficiently as possible with the highest bill. They're running a business, and many floors are understaffed and overworked. A C-section is simply the fastest way to get the baby out. It seemed that women's overall well-being was not a priority for our broken system. Even things like pain management during invasive, painful procedures were standard practice in men's healthcare, but not in women's.

They described in detail how painful their experiences were and how they wish they'd known to ask for pain meds. I compared that with stories of men getting a vasectomy. The procedure is always done under a minimum of local anesthesia, while some are put under sedation sometimes based upon patient preference. They are then often prescribed narcotic pain meds afterward. Many women describe only receiving Tylenol after even a C-section.

I couldn't seem to get any of the midwives to tell me what I wanted to hear, which was "You won't have to have one!" Although I had a healthy pregnancy, and my baby was in the proper position for vaginal delivery, birth is unpredictable. Because of this, I'd heard that some women even opt-in for an elective C-section.

"I loved my C-section!" Connor's mom said.

Some women and/or their doctors prefer the controllable and predictable nature of it being scheduled. For high-risk pregnancies, it often is the safest option. It's the unknown and release of control that scares many of us about labor. C-sections do come with their own risks as major surgeries, but at least it's in the doctors' hands.

I'd never had surgery. It scared me to my core. Being awake for one? I could not and would not do it.

24 Cascade of Interventions

"Maternity care in the United States is intervention intensive," one article began from the Natural Library of Medicine by Judith A. Lothian. "These interventions disturb the normal physiology of labor and birth and restrict the women's ability to cope with labor. The result is a cascade of interventions that increase the risk of cesarean surgery for women and babies."

There it was all in writing. Scholarly sources like this backed up the scary stories I had seen warning me of this "Cascade of Intervention," that evidently was the path that led American women to the operating room. Intervention typically refers to procedures doctors use to assist or expedite the baby's exit. A common one was induction. I hadn't heard of this before.

"How long do you think you can stand being this pregnant?" one of the midwives smiled as she asked me at my 38-week appointment. I liked her. She was an older woman with long gray hair and looked like she'd been doing this for a while. I trusted her. I hoped she'd be the one who would deliver Claire when the time came. Hospitals typically have you see a variety of practitioners on a rotating basis, rather than just one. I always thought it would be one person the whole way through, but they said it's to ensure I'm comfortable with everyone since they can't predict who would be on shift that day when I'd go into labor.

"I'd like to give birth today!" I laughed, not yet that her question was literal.

"When would you like to be induced?" she asked, more seriously.

"Induced… Oh. Well, when do you typically do it?" I asked, wishing I'd read more on my own before the appointment. Usually, they just checked my blood pressure and I'd be on my way. My stomach dropped as I noticed this appointment was different because I'd actually have to get this baby out of my body soon.

"We don't recommend going past your due date. What do you think about 41 weeks? She suggested, sensing my nerves.

"I guess I can't imagine going much further. I'm really in pain, like everywhere." I replied.

I'd made similar complaints to another midwife at the appointment a week earlier. My belly was gigantic at 37 weeks. I struggled carrying the sheer weight of it as I walked. I hobbled and waddled through Magee Hospital, wincing with every few steps into their office. On one particularly long stretch of hallway overlooking the Oakland area of Pittsburgh, I felt a tearing right above my belly button, where I'd been feeling pain all week. My ab muscles had split open.

"Thank God I'm at the hospital," I thought.

The young and cool-girl midwife walked in and shut the door. I was relieved to see it was her. She had a septum piercing and looked about my age. I felt comfortable with her because she'd done a pap smear for me earlier in the pregnancy. She was the gentlest health professional to this day to ever touch me. She went slowly and walked me through each touch after seeing how anxious I was. I hated the feeling of all these strangers messing with my cervix something so deep inside my body it seemed it was never designed to be touched. I shook every time my feet hit the stirrups.

"How are you feeling?" she asked, sitting down to take notes in her computer.

I sat on the table, assuming she'd rush me to the ER downstairs when I told her.

"I think my abs have torn open. I literally felt it on the way here. It hurts so bad. It feels like my torso will split open completely!"

I waited for her to match my shock, but she barely looked up from the computer. She nodded.

"By this point in the pregnancy, everything is very uncomfortable," she said.

She said Diastasis Recti is what I was feeling, and that my abs had in fact split open. I could stick my fingers in between them and physically see the gap in the muscles on my belly. Apparently, it's normal, and yet another thing pregnant women never discuss that, to me, seemed like a huge deal.

This must be why women agree to inductions, I thought, for the relief.

Inductions Crash Course

I dove into inductions, the how, the why, the side effects, and how the body naturally goes into labor without one.

Despite most hospitals suggesting induction at 38 weeks, first-time moms on average go into labor around 41 weeks and 5 days gestation naturally, and it's all powered by hormones. I was sick of hearing about them. Aren't you? All I'd known of hormones was that they were invisible magic vibes that dictate how our bodies operate. I learned they drive each stage of pregnancy, and they also would initiate when my body would go into labor, the primary one being Oxytocin.

I knew of Oxytocin as the "love hormone" that I'd always heard attached women to men after sex. It's much more. We also release it when we're relaxed and in a positive mindset. Midwives and doulas online recommended massages, sex, hugging, cuddling, dimmed lights, and relaxation to help the body produce it and initiate labor. Notice how conference meetings and Microsoft Teams calls are not listed there? Eliminating stress was the most important step because they all said the body can't produce enough oxytocin to go into labor naturally if stress hormones pumped through the body instead.

Inductions typically start with a vaginal insertion medication, usually Cytotec or Cervidil, to soften and/or help to dilate the cervix. Then, they administer Pitocin intravenously. My laymen's terms understanding of Pitocin was that it's a synthetic version of Oxytocin. It forces the uterus to contract, but more intensely than natural contractions. It forces labor on a body resisting it.

As a working mom, I knew Cortisol raged through *my* body like an electrical current, blockading the necessary Oxytocin. I'm in fucking sales, I thought. I enjoyed it, but stress is a normal part of the job. "Welcome to the show," we'd used to say to new hires the first time they cried on the job. I read numerous anecdotes about how modern working women like me struggle to go into labor on their own because they're expected to work until labor begins. If they're in a constant state of fight or flight, powered by Cortisol, blocking Oxytocin, natural labor seems unlikely. This made sense to me as to why inductions had become so common in the US. I wanted to let my body naturally go into labor on its own, avoiding the Cascade of Intervention but how, without an induction? I was determined to try.

25 The Sweep

We can't force labor without consequences or risks, yet it seemed modern women don't have time to allow their bodies to go into labor naturally. It was clear that I was on tight schedules, the schedules of my job and of the hospital network, and I'd better hurry. At work, people followed up with me daily as if my baby was an assignment nearing deadline. "Any update on when you'll be leaving or coming back?" My anxiety was already heightened, and my only answer to them was "I don't know," which never sufficed.

This most personal thing I'd ever experienced now felt so corporate. Childbirth is so sacred, and I believed my body should be allowed to do it at its own pace, not the pace of any board of stakeholders. Science does not fully understand labor yet, so why do we mess with it with so many interventions that have such high risks for the mother and baby? I wondered. Why do all roads seem to lead to C-section in so many hospital births? It's the quickest way for the hospital to get women out of the bed, and it seemed that was what the healthcare system wanted. There was a waiting list of women on call, waiting for the next bed, and my hospital was after all, "The baby factory." It was a name I originally thought was cute but now felt dystopian. The birth professionals and women I followed warned how to fight back against forced inductions and the ways the healthcare system steers women into unnecessary interventions. It all felt almost predatory.

There are good reasons for inductions, though. If a baby cooks past 40-42 weeks, the placenta can't supply the baby with oxygen and nutrients as efficiently. The risk of still-birth increases beyond this point. It seemed like such a fine line between making sure the pregnancy doesn't go on too long yet isn't rushed beyond necessity.

At my 40-week appointment, I was so uncomfortable and starting to feel desperate. I decided to try my first cervical check and membrane sweep. A cervical check is when the doctor or midwife inserts her hand into the birth canal and sees how many fingers he or she can fit into the cervix. A coworker told me she bled for a while afterward from the forceful digging after her first. I wanted no parts of it. I had declined the optional cervical checks at previous appointments, not only out of fear, but because they can increase infection risk and are apparently not even indicative of labor.

"You can be 1cm dilated and go into labor tonight, or you can walk around 4cm dilated for a month," one midwife confirmed.

"So why even do them?" I asked.

"Some women just like to know, and if you were to go into labor today, it's a starting point of reference," she said.

A membrane sweep was the last-ditch effort medical intervention before an induction. The doctor or midwife inserts their hand into the birth canal, shoves one or more fingers into the cervix, and digs in a circular motion to separate the embryonic sac from the cervix. It's intended to persuade the cervix to dilate sooner, leading to labor. Dependent on how dilated the mother already is, it only works 50%-80% of the time. Like the cervical checks, it comes with risk. The cervix naturally is closed for a reason, and introducing bacteria can lead to infection for the baby and mother. If they were to accidentally break my water, they said they'd have to introduce labor right away to get the baby out. My once strong mindset to stick up for myself and my baby had weakened. I was desperate enough to try the sweep. Not only could it lead me closer to relief from my physical symptoms, but it would also relieve me from my grueling work schedule, I considered. I could barely string a sentence together or waddle to my laptop in the morning, and I have no recollection of accomplishing anything during the last trimester, yet, like most American working women, I was shackled to my job until I could go into labor. This membrane sweep could be my escape, I thought.

I knew Claire was head down and I could feel her low in my pelvis. The heavy pressure on the lower part of my body was uncomfortable at every second of every day. I never forgot she was there. It was as if I'd swallowed a huge dumbbell and my pelvic floor was holding it like a hammock ripping slowly at its seams. The midwives assured me the sweep could be "uncomfortable, but not painful." Women's stories told me very much otherwise. TikTok was full of comment sections of women detailing traumatic pain. I read through hundreds of women agreeing, "The membrane sweep and cervical checks hurt worse than my natural birth with no epidural." My hands shook on the steering wheel on the way to the appointment.

"Let's see where this baby is!" the midwife said. I watched her hands as she stretched on her gloves and noticed her blue gel manicure that was about to be several inches inside me. I was grateful to see that her nails were short and shuddered at the thought of them digging around.

"Will this hurt? Be honest with me," I said gripping Connor's hand and lifting my feet onto the stirrups.

She sighed. "It's very uncomfortable." She lowered her voice. "If this were men's healthcare, they'd have found a less invasive and painless way to do this, right?"

I locked my eyes on the drop ceiling and pulled Connor's hand closer, bracing myself.

"Here we go," she said like this was about to be a treacherous expedition.

I felt her hand stretch and tear into me and felt her nails dig into my cervix. Her finger stabbed and grinded as she lightly grunted with the physical force.

"You're doing good," Connor said wiping my tears and squeezing my hand until it stopped.

I slowed my breathing as I watched her remove her slightly bloodied glove.

"You are not dilated at all," she said. "I couldn't get in far enough for the sweep. I'm sorry, but remember, you could come back here in two hours and be 4cm dilated! You just never know!"

I couldn't believe I endured that pain and violation in vain. I felt I was doing this all wrong, and it was my fault that I wasn't at least 1-2cm dilated. I worried I'd be pregnant forever, and an induction seemed more likely.

26 My Induction

I waved my white flag and agreed to the induction. Most first-time mothers go into labor naturally at an average of 41.5 weeks, despite the pressure to do it earlier. I felt that all my hard work to go into labor naturally had failed. At 41 weeks, the induction was scheduled for tomorrow, but that didn't mean we got a specific time. We had to wait for a bed to open.

"We'll call you within a 24-hour period between 12AM tonight and 12AM tomorrow night," the nurses told me on the phone.

"So, we need to just be ready to leave at the drop of a hat for 24 hours?" I asked.

"Correct." The anticipation was mental torture. I felt more than nervous. It was pure, primal fear.

Would I survive childbirth? Would my baby survive? What if Connor had to tell the doctor which one of us to save? If I do survive, will I tear down through my asshole or upward through my... I can't even go there.

My mind raced as I curled my hair in the bathroom mirror that evening before bed. My hands were so swollen they could barely close to wrap around the curling iron and each squeeze felt like my fingers would burst open, but I wanted to look pretty for birth. I'd have Connor or a nurse take photos of me with our fresh new baby on my chest. I don't even go to the grocery store without makeup on, and this was my big moment, one I'd remember forever. It was hard for me to feel pretty at all, so I figured curling my hair and packing my makeup would at least make me feel less like Shrek and a bit more like Fiona.

In these last few weeks, I'd looked so forward to not being pregnant, to feel relief from the pain, but now I wanted to be pregnant longer. Finally, around 10PM, I turned HGTV off, tried to do some breath work for calming anxiety, and turned my phone on loud, knowing the hospital could call overnight when I least expected it. Suddenly at 10:30PM, earlier than planned, my phone rang. It woke me in a panic like an alarm alerting a community to impending natural disaster.

"Hi Katie? I'm a nurse at Magee Hospital. We should have a bed for you right at midnight. Can you get here soon?"

I rushed downstairs to Connor. "They're ready for us." I could barely get the words out.

"Already?" He shot up off the couch.

One benefit of the induction is that we were, although scared, mentally prepared for at least some sort of timeframe. Our bags were packed and ready on the dining room table, one for us and one for Claire. Hers was soft and cream-colored with tiny little teddy bears. It was filled with tiny onesies and a few "going home" outfit options with matching hats and bows. Ours had an extra comfy outfit, a cute outfit for pictures for me, phone chargers with extra-long cables to stretch around the room, recommended by our parent-veteran friends.

Walking into Magee in the middle of the night felt surreal. The usually bustling crowded hospital was dark and quiet. I looked up at Connor as we held hands walking into the lobby.

"When we walk out of this building, we'll be a family of 3," I said.

He kissed my hand, "I know."

We both yawned, and I couldn't believe we were expected to begin this journey in the middle of the night. We were already exhausted, and we hadn't even started yet.

Inductions are so popular that they had their own unit so that the processes could be monitored and controlled differently than those of women in spontaneous labor. In 2019, CDC data showed that almost a quarter of American labors are induced, having increased steadily since the 90s, when it was under 10%. This little room was cozy, as much as a hospital room can be. It had a recently renovated private bathroom with a shower and a couch bed for Connor. I tried not to get too comfortable because I knew I'd spend time here just in the beginning until I was dilated enough to graduate to the Labor & Delivery Floor. I wondered I'd be here 30 minutes or 3 hours.

There are typically two induction medications used to initiate women into labor, Cytotec and Cervidil. Cervidil is usually administered vaginally, and Cytotec can be given either vaginally or orally. I'd heard about them on TikTok. I was so nervous I forgot to ask which one they were using on me before the midwife's whole fist was in there. I wished I had the information and the choice as to how we went about this. It knocked the wind out of me, just like the membrane sweep. She shoved a few tiny pills in there.

"They're in! Now we wait," she said. It was the midwife I'd hoped for. I was glad to see it was her who'd deliver my baby, and I felt comforted as soon as I saw her long gray hair and heard the familiar voice coming down the hallway. A young nurse named Samantha came in with a clipboard and gently exposed my belly. With her sweet, chill demeanor, this was all routine to her.

"Sorry, I'll take these off. They're silicon pads to prevent stretch marks," I said, making room for whatever she was about to do.

"Oh yeah, do they work?" she asked.

"No." I smiled as I gestured toward the purple wound-like stretch marks covering the bottom half of my belly.

She strapped my torso tightly bands that held heartrate monitors in place ever so perfectly positioned. I looked down at them and tried to imagine Claire scrunched up in there, orienting where her bum and belly must be based upon the monitor locations. I started to feel more ready as her big debut inched closer. Maybe by morning she'd be here, snuggled in my arms while I sipped a cappuccino from the coffee shop downstairs, I thought.

"Try to relax and get some sleep. You're going to need it!" Samantha said.

I turned slightly to my side to be able to rest my head on the familiar pillow behind me that Connor brought from home for me. Within minutes, Samantha came running into the room fiddling with the monitors. Her face, once pleasant and calming, was wide-eyed with focus, and she had a serious, stern tone to her voice.

"What's wrong?" I said groggily. Connor was sound asleep on the couch.

"The baby's heartrate dropped. Turn on your other side, now! All the way," She instructed me before finally exhaling. I'm pretty sure my heart stopped in the process. I looked at her speechless.

"It's alright. All good now," she said, but I hadn't yet taken a breath. She could tell I didn't believe her yet.

"I'm not worried. Sometimes babies can't handle certain positions when they're this far along. She was probably lying on her cord. Just don't turn on that side anymore," she said.

After that scare, I was too afraid to take a deep breath let alone move from the exact position she put me in. I watched the clock go from 12AM to 6AM in what felt like minutes. It was Monday, and maybe today would be the day I'd meet Claire, I thought! I was trying to erase the work-related Monday thoughts from my brain when the midwife came back in with one of her peers, one of the few I hadn't met yet.

"I'll be taking over for you," she said with a kind tone touching my leg. The midwives had great bedside manner, and I needed their gentle tones more than I thought I would. I was so disappointed that my favorite midwife was leaving. I didn't think that the world was moving outside this room and that when the clock was ticking, hours were actually passing by. These were just people finishing their work shifts, and there wouldn't be one common voice with me from start to finish.

The new midwife was younger with long pretty, blonde hair. She and the new nurses prepared me for my next cervical check to see how dilated I'd gotten. I felt like I was being graded on my performance or achievement.

"I know these have been hard for you, and that's normal. Let me know if we need to stop. I should tell you that the hormones in the medicine we put in there do make the area much more sensitive, so this may be a lot more uncomfortable than the ones before," she said as the nurse planted her feet steady on the floor and grabbed my hand like we were about to take off into flight. There was that word again, "uncomfortable." I knew what she meant. I returned the nurse's grip and braced myself. I heaved through the pain and tried not to scream, which seemed impolite. She was right. It was way more intensely painful, yes painful not "uncomfortable." There's nothing else on earth to compare it too, but I imagine being impaled with a steak knife should suffice. I felt nauseous. As she exited me, we were both sweating and breathless.

"I can't feel anything," she said with a disappointed look. I'd failed, I thought.

My mind said, "Are you fucking kidding me," as my mouth said, "What?"

"Your cervix is still pretty closed. You're at about 2cm. I think we do more of the medicine," she said. In again she went. This cyclical routine of torture went on all day and into the night. Every few hours they'd lower the bed backward, and I'd brace myself for the pain.

"You told me you struggled with these, but you did great," the next nurse on shift said.

"Most women scream super loud, but you got through it with some mostly heavy breathing. That's impressive!" She congratulated me, and I did hear my peers screaming around the hallway like a Halloween haunted house. Since the checks are routine, hospitals typically don't offer pain relief medication, but midwifery blogs recommend certain tricks like a cough or deep breath to ease into it. I wished I was more mentally prepared for all of it.

27 Labor Day 2

Time kept moving outside the induction floor, but because I hadn't slept, I barely noticed. I only knew how long exactly by the dates on the calendar because it was like time stopped. I had no conceptualization of the outside world and didn't care. Everyone kept telling me to sleep, but I was in too much pain and still traumatized from violence of the cervical checks. People know that the actual birth will hurt. Women have heard of that by now as humans, but no one told me about all the things leading up to the birth that were also extremely painful.

The contractions had also started. It was gradual. At first, I just felt my belly tightening, and I could see it squeeze, then release after about a minute. It was uncomfortable and strange to not be in control of what felt like my entire torso, but it wasn't painful.

"It's happening! I'm doing it!" I said to Connor, pointing to my tensing belly-sphere.

As the hours progressed, the pain grew bit by bit, and it felt similar to a bad menstrual cramp. I was actually excited to feel contractions because it meant I was progressing, and finally, I was doing something right.

Monitoring

One of the tight bands on my belly was tracking the contractions and showed them rising and falling on a graph monitor next to the hospital bed. It had my heart rate, the baby's heart rate, and the contractions all on one screen. I was fascinated watching the line climb into a hill as my belly tightened, then relaxed. It reminded me again that I was merely an observer and passenger. Nature and my body were in control.

How the hospital monitors the baby is another protocol that differs from hospital to hospital. There are two most common methods. There is continuous external monitoring, during which the monitors are attached to the belly the whole time, or there is intermittent monitoring. During intermittent monitoring, they check the heartrate about every 30 minutes during active labor, and every 5 minutes during pushing, according to Kaiser Permanente's website.

It seemed most healthcare networks, organizations, and researchers agreed that intermittent monitoring was better for low-risk pregnancies.

"You're not attached to monitors all the time, so you can move about more freely. It can help reduce the use of labor interventions and can lower the chances of a Cesarean," Kaiser Permanente's website continued in a 2022 article.

Although this seemed a wide-spread understanding in the medical community, many hospitals, including mine, opt for continuous monitoring as standard protocol, even for low-risk patients.

The monitor bands were so tight around me and had been stuck in the same position for two days now. From these being pressed into me for so long, my right kidney was in intense pain. I couldn't move or adjust because if I did, they'd lose the signal of the heartbeat and need to correct the placement.

"I need to move around," I told the nurse. "I heard laying and sitting still is the worst thing I can be doing for labor, and I haven't been progressing. I'm going to walk around the halls," I finally demanded.

"Okay we'll have to use wireless monitors then," the nurse told me. I wondered why this wasn't an option they'd mentioned outright.

I resented that the nurses and midwives knew what would help me progress faster, yet encouraged me to do the opposites. The TikToks were right. I'd have to fight for myself and my baby. I'd learned in birthing class, and of course on TikTok, that the toilet is "the dilation station." Sitting backward on the seat would allow gravity to help me dilate more quickly. L&D nurses and doulas online all swore by this. Squatting, walking and moving in general is the best thing to do in order to progress. I knew that this was why the Epidural slows labor, often leading to a c-section, and remembered the "cascade of intervention." I was determined not to fall victim to it. I huffed and puffed and waddled up and down the hallway for hours, sitting on the "dilation station" in between. Walking helped ease the contraction pain, which at this point felt like horrible menstrual cramps.

The nursing supervisor came in to ask how my experience with my nurses had been.

I wasn't going to go off on a tangent about my thoughts on US healthcare and how the nurses should be trained to better progress labor, in my opinion, rather than keeping me in bed to be closer to the c-section, so I digressed. It didn't seem the time or place for a system-wide criticism. Maybe I was afraid of tattling on the nurses. Maybe I was so tired that I just didn't have it in me to take on the hospital. I didn't want to be a bother. I was stuck here and needed the nurses to like me so that they'd treat me and my baby well. I felt in their mercy and figured I shouldn't piss them off.

"Everything's been fine," I said, "Just excited to meet the baby and hoping this speeds up soon. The contractions really don't even hurt that badly. It's bearable!"

She laughed. "Hold onto that feeling, honey. You'll need it!"

28 Labor Day 3

"We're moving you to the L&D Floor!" My nurse
hurried in.

"Oh sweet! This means you think the baby is going to
come today? Things are further along?" I asked, in more
pain now, as the contractions have gotten stronger.

"No, we just need this bed," she said, "But they'll start
your Pitocin, and things should pick up from there."

Feeling embarrassed that I'd overstayed my welcome,
Connor and I packed up and I walked to the elevator and
through the halls to the new room. I had no idea if it was
day or night. Walking into our new room, I took in every
detail. This was the room where I'd meet my baby. It had a
bigger bathroom with outdated tile that smelled like pee but
had plenty of room. The overall room was huge compared
to the induction room. The lights were off, and it was quiet.
It must be nighttime, I thought. Connor yawned. I waddled
to my new hospital bed. Across from me was a tiny static-
filled TV and a little plastic bassinet. I imagined, for the
millionth time, the moment when Claire would come out
from between my legs, and I'd pull her close to my chest
with tears of joy and Connor at my side. Then they'd place
her in that exact bassinet. I pictured her wrapped up in there
like a little pastry with the little pink and blue blanket and
hat the hospital always uses. She'd be in there soon. The
vision I'd been excited for all year would finally happen
right here in this room. By this point, I hadn't slept in more
than two days and was completely exhausted. I could tell
my body needed rest. Although I wasn't purposefully doing
much, my body was contracting and in labor, working

around the clock. I was so sick of this waiting. I tried my best to move around, squatting, walking, sitting on the toilet and got excited every time I saw bloody mucus come out. The mucus plug seals the cervix shut and when it comes out in a "bloody show" it can be a sign of labor progressing as the cervix dilates. Toward the end of my third trimester, I looked eagerly for it every time I found myself in the restroom but never saw it until I was deep in labor. Like the contractions, I was excited to feel the progress and knew I was one step closer to meeting my baby.

Breaking Water

The midwife came in for another hellish cervical check, and when she did, I felt a small flow of what felt like pee streaming out of the wrong hole.

"Oh, I feel fluid coming out! I think my water broke!" I was embarrassed that I couldn't control this bodily fluid spewing all over this fresh bed. "Sorry," I said to her and the nurse.

"Don't apologize. This is exciting," she said as she prepared her fist.

I writhed in the familiar pain. "Your water did break, but the sac is still intact. It must have broken at the top and is trying to get out around the head. We'll need to break the rest for you," she said, reaching for a long plastic hooked needle I couldn't fathom going anywhere near where I knew it was going.

She broke the sac further all over the towels the nurse had tucked under me, and I noticed how different this was than the movies. You always see a woman going about her day when *SPLASH* Her water breaks onto the sidewalk and she rushes to the hospital, giving birth in what seems like minutes. This felt less exciting and nowhere near magical, but I thought we'd gotten this show on the road. Now, we'd wait for my cervix to cooperate and dilate further.

IV bags ran through me routinely. When we had that first heartrate scare when I first arrived, they began to flood me with fluid. They told me it was to fill my amniotic sac enough to give the baby room to move around. If it's too empty, the pressure could compress the cord and she'd lose oxygen quickly, which we'd already caught once. The fluid made me swell even more. By this point, even my eyelids were so engorged that my eyes were nearly swollen shut. My legs and arms looked like tree trunks. I didn't care what I looked like anymore. At least my hair was curled, but it was greasy now since I'd been here for days longer than I anticipated. My neatly packed makeup bag was nowhere in sight. The other IV was antibiotics. I'd tested positive for strep B. In the third trimester, they shove a Q-Tip in your rear-end to test for it. A third of women have it at the time of birth, and it can be fatal if it touches the baby's fresh skin. Antibiotics during labor prevents it.

"Okay girl, this honestly is going to really burn. Here's a heating pad. It helps," a nurse told me as she put it in. "Ask the next nurse for one too. This is where they hide them."

Finally, someone was being real with me. She was right about the antibiotics. It burned like hell. That IV was connected to a vein in my wrist. I looked robotic with all the tubes coming in and out of me like exposed electrical wiring on a bionic character in a sci-fi movie. I could feel the medicine burn all the way through my forearm. The heating pad did help, and I asked each new nurse for one. None of them offered, and I was grateful the first nurse looked out for me even after her shift ended.

A while after my water was broken, I was about 5cm dilated. Halfway there. I knew I'd push at 10cm, and the real show would begin. The room was dark.

Support Person

It's recommended that women have a "support person," if not a professional doula in the room during labor. They're there to remind the mom to breathe through pain and offer words of encouragement. In our birth class, the instructor showed us massages they can do to help moms with the lower back pain of labor. I figured my support person would be Connor by default, but I don't think he had any concept of how to actually support me. He wasn't seeing me screaming and cussing like women do in the movies, so I think he thought that labor hadn't truly begun. The secret about labor is that it's not like those movie scenes. For many like me, it's a tortuously long process, taking, in my case, several days.

Connor had been asleep for hours. He's known for sleeping anywhere. In our twenties, I'd walk into a loud house party with his DJ friends blasting dubstep and find him sound asleep on the couch next to the speaker. Put him in a warm and cozy room with dimmed lighting, and the guy is doomed. I was a little annoyed that he was peacefully slumbering through this, but I was grateful I was able to mentally process everything in solitude. My therapist had always told me, "You process your emotions alone before taking them to others and that's okay." Plus, this was one lengthy uneventful hospital stay so far. He tried to stay awake, but the calm and dark room lulled him right to sleep the whole time. Everything was happening so slowly that I think he forgot I was in labor.

I remembered in my birthing class that the instructor mentioned the L&D nurses would be putting me in all different positions and giving me various contraptions to try to get the baby out and help me progress. I was disappointed to find that I didn't have that experience at all. I saw my L&D nurses seldomly, and they didn't say much unless I asked them something, which I didn't do often for fear of bothering them. I repeatedly told them I wanted to "labor down," but that I didn't know how. They didn't really respond, and they left me in bed.

"You good?" Connor asked me, waking up to go pee. He yawned.

"No. This is starting to get real," I said as I paced and rocked back and forth in the dark, trying to breathe through the contractions.

It felt like the worst menstrual cramp of all time on top of the worst stomachache from diarrhea all at once, covering my belly all the way into my back. I was sweating and shaking a little. Staying still felt like hell. I had to move through the pain. I remembered that growing up my mom used to always tell me to walk when I had cramps from my period.

"I know you want to lay down, but that makes it worse. Move!" she'd urge me as I groaned and peeled myself off the couch.

I barely noticed as Connor walked past me and went right back to sleep. I could feel the weight of the baby on the bottom of my spine like there was an elephant stepping on it. I wondered if it would disintegrate from the pressure.

It might be better if it just crumbled and got out of the way, I thought.

Resisting the Epidural

I was so afraid to ask for the epidural even though I knew it would stop most of the pain. I remembered what I'd heard about asking too early, but I also heard anecdotally not to ask for it too late.

"Make sure you ask for the epidural like two hours BEFORE you've reached your limit, not after you've reached it," my friend Jacqueline's husband told me a few months ago.

I never forgot the way they told their birth story with their son. Connor jokingly referred to their birth as "The Great War." Jacqueline was in labor for three days, which looked a lot like where I was headed. Her doctor urged her to concede and accept a C-section from the first day onward, but she refused, knowing her baby's heartrate was fine. While she was pushing, her doctor noticed she was tearing and gave her an episiotomy, cutting her to the side to prevent tearing in a worse direction. She persisted through the gore and eventually pushed out her 10-pound son.

"I'm sorry I doubted you," her doctor told her.

"I watched Jacqueline reach her limit with the Pitocin contractions in hell, finally ask for the epidural, only for them to take like 2 hours to show up with it." her husband said. "So my theory is, ask for it when you think you're almost at your limit, like 60% there. That way, they show up with the epidural right on time when you're about to lose it."

I liked this theory, but being my first time at this, I had no idea how to gauge my "limit." Pain tolerance is relative to each person. In general, I always hate when doctors ask us "What's your pain on a scale of one to ten?" I find that hard to answer, not knowing what we're considering the ten, being burned alive? Should that make my sore throat a three? If I saw a number too low will I not get the same urgency or care?

At this point in labor, I was in agony and nauseated from the pain. Was that it, my limit?

"I really want a natural birth. I do not want a C-section, so let me know what I can do in your experience," I said over and over to each nurse with each shift change, assuming they'd have a plan of things to try. I knew they had a whole closet of tools that I learned about in the birthing class. They had poles and bars that somehow hook onto the hospital bed, long pieces of fabric to pull on or wrap around a woman's back, bouncing balls, and peanut balls. To ask for these seemed like ordering off the secret menu at Chipoltle or Starbucks. It was an inconvenience and a secret, as if this was some speakeasy where you needed to know the password or code to have a good time. They all just stayed mostly silent and didn't offer any suggestions. I couldn't remember what anything was called except the peanut ball, so I asked for that.

"Um yeah, let me see if I can find one," the nurse said.

I wished I'd had a doula

I regretted not having one. Everyone on social media warned me this might be the case, but I didn't want to have another big financial expense. I wasn't sure how much the hospital bill would be, but I knew it would be at least a few thousand dollars for a basic, healthy birth. It ended up being about $7,000 after insurance. My local doula network prices were tiered. Tier I was $1,250 and included more junior doulas who'd assisted in only 4-10 births. Tier II doulas had done 11-50 births and charged $1,500, and Tier III doulas with 51+ births charged $1,900. Doula services and prices vary, but common offerings include help with creating a birth plan and advocating with your provider for it, emergency on-call availability, labor support, and postpartum care. I figured I'd taken the class, read the books, watched the videos… I'd know exactly what to do. I didn't. In the exhaustion, I lost the information I'd learned and the confidence I'd built. It was like showing up to the SATs after 5 days of no sleep and starvation, set up for failure, no matter how hard I studied. All that I remembered was to hold off on the epidural as long as I could, but not too long to where I'd be unbearably suffering.

Pain Management

I called the quiet nurse who didn't say much into the room, and about 20 minutes later she appeared.

"You okay?" she asked.

"I think so, but I need something for the pain, please. I'm so exhausted I haven't slept. I'm just hoping I can take a nap to prepare for pushing. Everyone keeps telling me I'll need my energy. I don't want the epidural yet because I know it slows labor, and I've already progressed so slowly."

"You should just get the epidural. It works the best," she said.

"What about the gasses or IV meds? Tell me about those, please," I said, and I could tell I was annoying her by not letting her contain me to the hospital bed on the epidural. She must have been busy tonight.

"The gas doesn't really take away pain. It just makes you feel high so you're more comfortable handling it," she explained, referring to the nitrous oxide gas. "Some girls say it just makes you feel like you're still in the same amount of pain, but you're floating."

"Okay maybe… What else?" I pressed her.

"We could try Nubane. It's in an IV. It helps the pain temporarily, but it can make you feel really drunk so you won't be able to go to the bathroom alone for a while. You'll be super dizzy. You really should consider the epidural," she urged.

"Let's do the Nubane. I'm cool with feeling drunk, as long as I feel numb enough to take a nap."

To me, the Nubane was fucking awesome. I felt euphoric. It was the first taste of respite I'd had in days. I was high, the pain was eased majorly, not gone, but enough for me to finally fall asleep. I didn't even realize how much pain I was actually in until it was suddenly gone. My hand and arm stung from the IV and antibiotics burning through my veins, the tight bands that had squeezed me like taught rubber bands all over my torso, my back and hip pain that I'd had since February, the migraine, all gone. In all my life, I'd never deprived myself of sleep and food like this. Letting my body and mind rest was such a relief. When I woke up after about an hour, the pain was back, everywhere, and I was dizzy. I was yelling at Connor to wake up, but he's such a heavy sleeper that no decibel would do the trick. I threw a pillow at him and missed. He snored. I hit my call button for the nurse because I had to pee, and at this stage in pregnancy, every pee was an emergency. I also learned in the birth class that emptying the bladder is important during labor so it's not in the way of the baby descending through the pelvis. At this rate, I needed my bladder as empty as possible. I was over being in labor. I didn't care if she ripped me in two coming out, I just wanted this to be over. For a moment, I let myself imagine the repose of death, but quickly pushed it out of my mind, afraid if I went there, I couldn't come back.

After about 20 minutes without the nurse, I was starting to pee myself and decided I was determined to make it to the bathroom. I grabbed onto my metal IV hanger with wheels on it to stabilize myself in the dark room. I thought I'd fall over, but I remembered I'd walked home drunk enough times to be proficient in wobbling. I also remembered my childhood Irish dance teacher, Sheila, telling us as children to remind ourselves, "I'm a dancer," when we'd start to lose our balance on one foot. For some reason, it grounded us. "I'm a dancer," I said with every slow step as I swayed forward on the hospital tile all the way to the bathroom. The nurse walked in on me struggling to stand off the toilet.

"Oh, thank God you're here," I said with an exhale. The bathroom was gross. The floor smelled like pee, and it was turning my stomach. "Can you help me back to bed, please? You were right about the Nubane. I feel so dizzy."

"Yeah, I actually can't believe you made it all the way into here by yourself," she said, with my IV in one hand and my arm in the other.

"Anyway, the pain is back fully, so can I have some more of that? It was helping me sleep and I just want to sleep so badly," I begged, speaking slowly through a painful contraction.

"Well, I need to talk to your midwife because your baby doesn't seem to like it," she said reluctantly, hoisting me back into bed.

I hated this child-like tone and language they all used with me when talking about something related to my baby, as if *I* was a baby too. Outside these walls, I was a respected, intelligent adult. I was a working professional, a property owner, a fully functioning member of society, but in here, I felt like a toddler. I wanted them to shoot it to me straight.

"Wait so her heart rate is still kind of up and down?" I asked her, trying to focus my eyes, still drunk from the Nubane.

"I'll have the midwife come and talk to you as soon as she can," she said, hoisting me back onto the bed, keeping her voice soft to not wake Connor. God forbid we disturb him.

I waited with anxiety and a stiff neck, rubbernecking to the left to stare at the heart monitor screens next to me. I wouldn't take my eyes off her heart rate, watching it fluctuate with each contraction. I was so worried.

"Hold on Claire. This is almost over," I said to my belly.

Finally, after about an hour, a midwife appeared, the one with the long pretty blonde hair. At the beginning of her shift, it was straight and smooth, clearly flat-ironed perfectly. Now it was knotted onto a frizzy mess on the top of her head. She came in removing her mask with her hands on her hips catching her breath and wiping sweat from her brow. She'd clearly been through some shit and was ready to go home.

"I'm sorry about the Nubane. Thank you for your patience. I got here as soon as I could when I heard you were struggling. We can't do any more pain meds because the baby doesn't like it," she said. There goes the toddler tone again.

"So, her heart rate isn't stable? Like she's in danger right now?" I asked in a serious adult tone to establish that I wanted them to cut the shit and get to the point.

"A lot of babies can't handle Pitocin. The contractions are very intense, and she's not handling them well. We don't like where her heart rate goes with each contraction, but we're still okay. It's just something to keep an eye on, and we don't want to risk anything further by giving you more medication that could affect her heartrate," she said.

"Alright. I don't want the epidural yet. I want to keep going. I really don't want to do a C-section," I reminded her, as she left and introduced the new shift's midwife on the way out.

29 Surrender

I looked at the dry-erase-marker on the white board facing the hospital bed that tracked my progress like a report-card of my performance. I read that I was at 6-7cm, and I now was in so much pain I was no longer thinking straight. It was as if I no longer existed, only pain and agony did. If my soul could have my body, it would have. Once again, as I thought with the cervical checks too, I didn't know this level of pain was possible for the human body. I hit my call button and rocked on my feet, groaning. Connor stretched and woke up as the nurse came in.

"I'm tapping out. Epidural," I said before she could get a word out.

I was relieved to see the anesthesiology team come in. A few of my friends had expressed concern that I was delivering at the university hospital, UPMC. It was known as one of the best hospitals in Pittsburgh, but it also meant that students were learning with the patients. They have to learn somehow, I thought.

"You know you can request that you don't want any students to touch you, only to observe," a nurse friend said at dinner one night.

"But then you might need to wait 3 hours for the actual anesthesiologist to come in like I did," another friend chimed in.

I always figured I'd request the actual anesthesiologist and just do it early enough in case I needed to wait for them. Well, I'd waited too long. I couldn't wait any longer, and I'd have done it myself at this point.

"I'm one of the residents here, and this is one of our medical students," the resident said. They were both young men, probably a little younger than me. "He won't touch you, but I'm teaching him if it's okay with you for him to watch?"

"I don't care just please help me," I said, barely able to speak. The words came out one at a time with labored breath in between.

He and Connor helped me sit up on the edge of the bed, bending me slightly over my belly so my back was rounded and stretched. I groaned and wailed in pain.

"I know it's hard, but it's important that you stay very still," he said. "We're going to numb you. This will be a big, big pinch."

Don't you hate when doctors say something will be a "pinch?"

As I felt the needle graphically go into my spinal area, I cried in pain. I could see tears welling in Connor's eyes. He'd never seen me like this. I was always the calm in our storms, and I was broken. I'd played off the rest of the experience thus far and kept a smile for him so as not to scare him, but I'd now given up.

"Okay, you made it through the hard part. You should be numb now, and you shouldn't feel this second part," the resident said.

I exhaled, relieved… until BAM I felt what I thought was a knife stab deep into my spine. I screamed and shrieked, thinking he had stabbed me and was trying to kill me. If that was the needle, surely something was very wrong. I thought I'd now die. This pain was violent. How could someone do something like this to me? I wiggled my feet to make sure I wasn't paralyzed. I thought I was supposed to feel safe in a hospital, and I'd now been hurt by every person I'd met here, this being the worst.

"Oh, my bad!" the resident said, which is not what anyone wants to hear as they're playing with their spine. I held back vomit, not wanting to make a mess on the floor.

"You weren't supposed to feel that. I should have checked if you were numb. Have you ever needed extra numbing at the dentist?" he asked.

Everyone's bodies react differently to these medications, and even genetics can play a part. For example, I later read that something as random as having red hair can mean someone needs more anesthesia for it to be effective. I remembered I did need more numbing shots when I got a root canal years ago, but I couldn't respond. I was sobbing in pain. I was done. I was past my limit of endurance for any more pain or any more strangers touching me, yet here came more contractions. He wrapped up and left the room as the nurse cleaned up the bloody mess and laid me back on the bed as I shook.

"The pain should start to ease now," she said, trying to comfort me.

I couldn't believe this was my epidural experience. Everyone had warned me about the "ring of fire" when the baby is crowning as the worst pain, but no one warned me about the pain of the epidural. I thought the epidural was supposed to be the "easy" way, taking *away* pain, not causing it. I'd heard some women on TikTok joke that they wanted to marry their anesthesiologist. I felt like no one would take this seriously and understand that I was traumatized by this. I thought I must have been the only one to experience this since the epidural was so great for everyone else. I must just be weak or have lower pain tolerance. It was my fault. I felt so alone. I didn't know then that epidural complications and pain are common. All I knew then was that this was a traumatic event I'd never forget.

"Wait, my peanut ball," I said to the nurse through the sobs as she rushed out of the room to her next patient .

I had to fight to get that damn thing in between my knees every time I moved. It was my last hope of progressing labor. I thought it was so strange as if they didn't want me to have it. I could tell it would be much easier on everyone if I just had a C-section; the nurses, the techs and medical assistants, the students, the midwives, Connor, and all our friends and family waiting for updates.

Again, I regretted not having a doula to fight for me when I couldn't fight for myself. I thought I'd be able to advocate for myself. I had no idea labor would break me down like this. The real me is strong, intelligent, and confident. She'd have no problem demanding what was best for me and my baby, but she was gone. It felt like they killed her, and I was a shell of who I once was. I understood now why they talked to me like a baby because they'd finally broken me down into one.

The epidural did relieve the pain, but only on one side of my body. I could still move my legs and feet. It felt like they were heavy and mostly numb like when your leg falls asleep and goes all tingly. Typically, they flip women from side to side every few hours so the medicine doesn't pool in one side of their back, but since Claire's heartrate dropped when I laid on my left side, I had to stay on my right. The medicine seemed to only work on that side. I pushed the button they gave me to release more, but I didn't notice a difference. It was still enough relief to fall asleep again.

30 The C-Section

A few hours later, after a nap and another savage fisting, I was at 8-9cm. I was almost ready to push at the 10cm finish line. Three days had passed since we'd walked into the hospital, and it was starting to feel like we'd never walk out of it. At 1AM, the midwife who'd done my failed membrane sweep appeared. Must be a new shift, meaning another 12 hours had passed, I thought. This was how I somewhat kept track of time and days passing. I noticed right away her short blue gel manicure and remembered feeling those same nails inside my cervix last week, digging for the membrane unsuccessfully as I winced and groaned. I felt sick. She came into the room and pulled up the chair next to the bed, something none of them had done yet. I knew something was off. She had bad news. I could see it in her furrowed brow and pitiful look in her eyes. The lights were still off, and Connor was sound asleep again for the night. I was too frozen to wake him up, so I braced myself to take this on alone for now, whatever it was.

"I need to talk to you about your baby," she said with her voice soft.

"We're at a crossroads. We need to give you more Pitocin to get you to push, but your baby hasn't been responding to it well. We've been watching her heartrate the last few hours while you slept. With each contraction, it drops, and we don't like to see that," she said, easing me into it, but I knew where this was going.

I stayed silent, too exhausted to respond. Her sitting there in the dark on the side of my bed reminded me of the way my mom would speak in the same soft tone, comforting me after a nightmare. I missed her and wished she was here. This had become a real-life nightmare, and there was no mom here to wake me up and save me. I was the mom now, and I was on my own.

"I'm not confident we can get her out safely without a C-section. If we push now and her heart rate drops, this becomes a much more serious situation. It's safer to do the C-section so we can better monitor and control her heartrate," she said, finally getting to the point she knew would hit me like a punch.

My heart sank deep into my chest and my breath disappeared like I'd been turned into stone. My nightmare I tried to evade from the moment I'd conceived caught me no matter how fast I'd run from it. I remembered seeing the pregnancy test in my bathroom last year, dreading this moment. How could this be? I worked so hard my entire 10-month pregnancy to ensure I could have a vaginal birth, fleeing from the statistics that all seemed to lead here. I hadn't sat back in my seat in 6 months to ensure the baby was in the right position. I'd done yoga poses and squats and considered acupuncture but had no more PTO to spend the time. It felt like the system had won, and I'd failed. I'd done everything I could to avoid this moment, and it still wasn't enough. I wondered what I'd missed and where I went wrong.

The heart rate monitor screen showing my heartrate climbed. I started to hyperventilate. "I can't," I said, starting to cry again. She held me in her arms.

"Oh my God. Connor's been asleep! I thought he was awake hearing this. Want me to wake him up?" I was too hysterical to respond to her.

"Connor!" she whisper-shouted to wake him up without scaring him too much.

Connor finally woke up, saw me in hysterics, and turned white as a ghost. "What's wrong?" he said, blinking hard to force his mind to wake up faster, scrambling off the couch.

"I have to get a fucking C-section," I sobbed. The midwife took over and told him about Claire's heartrate.

In a blur, I signed some paper on a clipboard. Seconds later, my bed was moving, and I saw the lights pass me on the ceiling as we rushed to the OR. Connor had to stay behind. I looked up at the anesthesiologist above my head on the way there. They'd brought in the big guns, no more residents or students.

"You do a lot of these everyday, right?" I asked, hoping she'd comfort me by telling me these are routine procedures and that everything would be easy for them. She didn't answer me, looking forward and focused. It was as though from this moment on, no one saw me, and they only saw my baby. I appreciated that she seemed on a mission to get my baby there and back alive.

The OR lacked the Zen ambiance of the dark labor and delivery room. It was bright and felt more sterile. It looked like I shouldn't see this room as a patient, like it was made for people who worked here the way that customers don't see the inside of the kitchen at a nice restaurant. The room was bustling. It was a crowd of new faces, the only familiar one being my midwife who, thankfully, stayed with me through the whole thing. She even remembered to grab my phone so she could take pictures for me. I emotionally clung to her and the stern anesthesiologist working above my head. She stayed there and was a constant focal point for me. I was afraid these could be my last moments, and I'd spend them in a room of strangers. I wanted Connor to be there so badly and had no idea where they'd left him.

"Hi, I'm one of the OR nurses with you today. How are you?" a new nurse said, in way too chipper of a tone like I was there to get my nails done.

"Terrified," I replied through the sobs. It was the only word I could muster when I wanted to say, "You're all about to slice me open and tear a human being out of my abdomen. How do you think I am, motherfucker?" Luckily for him, I couldn't string together a sentence.

"Aw," he said, offering nothing of comfort or reassurance.

I couldn't believe they were about to cut into my body essentially against my will, even though I wouldn't stop them. I knew we had to get this baby out, and I was out of options. The kicker is that I'd be awake for it. Patients are not awake or alert for any other major abdominal surgery. I tried to imagine the healthcare system telling men that they would need to be awake for a major and deep surgery of this caliber, or even a vasectomy. Not a shot in hell. I remembered the TikToks that I tried to scroll past but sometimes let myself watch for a little too long. They'd show women who could feel every part of their C-section, screaming on the table for the surgeon to stop or put them to sleep. I thought back to a Grey's Anatomy episode where a woman wakes up during a surgery after the anesthesia somehow failed. She could feel everything but was paralyzed, and she was psychologically ruined.

"Can you please put me under," I begged the midwife.

"No, unfortunately, it's better for the baby if you're awake, but we will numb you," she said.

A team of people appeared on either side of me. I tensed up, knowing something was about to go down.

"On the count of 3," the OR nurse muffled through his mask. Everyone suddenly grabbed the sheet under me like a hammock and swung me from my mobile hospital bed, where I'd spent the last day and a half, to the operating table. The seconds in the air were awful. I was so scared they'd drop me and felt helpless like livestock on its way to slaughter, alive, awake, fully sentient.

I landed on the table. I wasn't ready to die. They constructed a paper and sheet wall at my chest so I couldn't see anything that was happening to me beyond it.

"Try to be grateful that we have this option to save your baby," the surgeon said peeking over the sheet. I knew she was right. I imagined all the women throughout history who didn't have access to life-saving medical procedures like this.

A male doctor I assume was part of the anesthesiology team appeared above the sheet curtain.

"I'm going to take this object and move it down across your belly. You tell me when you stop feeling it." I stared at the bright light above the table and focused on a small pin-like object slowly dragging over the hump of my belly. It stopped around the equator of my bellybutton, demonstrating where I was numb.

"There," I said.

"Good. You tell us if you start to feel pain. You will feel movement, pressure, and pulling, but you shouldn't feel pain," he said. "Tell us if you do," he repeated.

Tools clinked around beyond the sheet wall. It sounded like a busy kitchen. As I listened and tried to translate their medical jargon-filled conversation, my body convulsed. I'd heard of "labor shakes," and only heard them described as a shiver. This was violent, and I was falling off the table. I had no control of my entire body. Every joint I had from my elbows to my jaw was possessed by some force, flailing my body parts around the table like a fish out of water. I worried and wondered how they'd hold the knife steady to cut me open. They pressed my arms down and out straight at my sides like I was being crucified. I thought it ironic because I was internally begging Jesus to get Claire and I both out of this room alive.

"Is this normal?" I asked them.

"Yes," they said as they covered my neck and shoulders with what looked like a big paper bubble. I looked like an inflatable Halloween costume with a head at the top. It reminded me of one year when Connor and I were inflatable Sumo wrestlers for Halloween. It was far from cozy and felt more like I was in a half-zipped body bag.

Finally, Connor appeared over the curtain and some relief poured over me. They'd gotten him into the whole get-up with a hair net, mask, and scrubs. He looked like he worked there. I could tell he was scared too. He sat on my right side and softly rubbed my arm as it still shook uncontrollably.

"It's okay, you're okay," he repeated, otherwise speechless.

"She's fine. It's just the medicine making her shake like this," the midwife told him.

I had no idea what was happening below the curtain, but I could feel them working on and around my belly. I imagined they were gathering all the scalpels and tools and disinfecting the area, preparing for surgery. I braced myself for the moment they'd cut into my body and wanted the suspense to end.

"Are you going to tell me when they start so I know what's going on," I looked up at the upside-down face of the anesthesiologist above my head.

"They started a while ago. They're working through the layers already. They're about halfway in," she said, absolutely shocking me. There was a team of people inside my bloodied torso, tearing and cutting open 7 layers into my body, yet I had no idea. The feeling of things moving around on top of my belly was them *inside* me.

I always thought that C-sections were quick, and I comforted myself by believing it would be over within a few minutes like a Brazilian wax. After a half-hour of cutting and no baby, I felt stuck in purgatory.

"How much longer?" "Are we almost done?" I repeated every few minutes like a restless child in the backseat of a minivan on a long road-trip.

Out of nowhere, a short baby's cry broke the silence. My eyes, that I'd had focused on the overhead light to keep me from panicking, darted to Connor as we gasped and looked at each other in shock. We both burst into tears. That was her voice. That was her, Claire. They lifted her up above the curtain just a bit to show me her face. I could only see her head above the curtain wall and through my eyelashes because my eyes were so swollen. She was soaked in my blood and her skin was purplish-blue. Her head was morphed into a crooked cone from being squeezed on her descent through my body. Her eyes were swollen shut. All I could do was cry. I'd never cried this much. Each moment was a new depth of pain and/or emotion I wondered how I could handle. In my magical vision of the birth of my baby, I yearned for the moment they'd place her on my chest to hold close to my heart. My detailed birth plan said I'd have the "golden hour" of skin-to-skin contact with her. I wanted her vernix to remain on her skin to help protect her from infection. I wanted delayed cord-clamping. I wanted Connor to cut the cord. I had it all mapped out and assumed I'd be able to advocate for these details. Instead, I laid helpless and paralyzed, convulsing and cut open on an operating table unable to see what they were doing to her as they rushed her away. I could only tell where they took her by the distance of her cries growing toward the left side of the operating room. I was relieved to hear her crying because it meant she was alive and breathing, but every fiber of me wanted them to bring her to me. I was angry. I felt robbed of this whole experience. I looked at the clock. 1:58AM.

"What's today's date?" I asked Connor, realizing I wasn't sure if it was still July or August yet. "August 8th. Wow, that's her birthday," he said, stroking my arm.

"She sounds great! She's got a good set of lungs on her," one of the nurses yelled over to us from the other side of the room. I imagined how scared Claire must be. She's never seen light before and these bright fluorescents probably burned her eyes. She was used to being safe and warm inside my body, listening to my voice, but now she was torn from me and moved across the room, which felt like miles away. She's probably so cold, I thought.

As I waited for them to bring her to me, I assume from the blood loss, my body went weak. I used the only energy I had left in me to stay awake. My eyes felt so heavy, and the room spun. I was nauseous. I felt the deepest pull to fall asleep, but how could I? I feared that if I let myself surrender, I'd never wake up. I still didn't know where Claire was.

"Is this normal? I feel like I'm going to pass out," I asked the familiar mask and hair net above my face, trusting her with my life but never learning her name.

"Yes, so now might be a good time to just take a nap," the anesthesiologist told me, as if my freshly born baby wasn't in the room on the biggest day of my life.

"We're almost done now, right?" I asked for the hundredth time, but sure now that we must be done. The baby was out. We did it, I thought.

"They're working on stitching you back up. It does take a long time because there are so many layers. You're about halfway through this," she said.

Halfway? I wanted to just die rather than endure this psychological torture chamber any longer. I imagined them shoving a needle and thread through every layer of my flesh.

Meeting my baby

"Here she is!" my midwife appeared with my phone, taking photos of us. I turned my head to the right toward Connor, and a nurse was holding my baby. Through the dizziness and sleepy fog, I saw her. Claire was swaddled in the typical blue and pink hospital blanket with a hat. She was quiet and looked at Connor wide-eyed. I was sad that she still hadn't seen a human face, only masks and poofy hair-nets in fluorescent lighting. The nurse gingerly passed her to Connor as he cried and had his magical moment that I knew I'd never get. I was still fighting the current pulling me toward unconsciousness. It was taking everything in me just to keep my eyes halfway open and keep my head turned in their direction. She stared at Connor with her lips pouted, not noticing me.

"Hi," was all he could say through his tears. His usually deep and strong voice was high-pitched and weak. I'd never seen him this delicate. It was beautiful.

"Touch her," he said, moving her close to my hand laid out at my side. I was still laid out like a cross.

My arms convulsed, but less violently now. I still had little control. I scrounged up the focus to lift my shaking hand and carefully let the back of my fingers stroke her cheek. I was heartbroken that I couldn't hold her, and we couldn't feel each other.

31 Recovery

I must have lost consciousness because my next
memory is being hoisted again off the table and onto
another mobile bed for transit to another wing of the
hospital. I yelped like an injured dog as they moved my
freshly sliced and sewn body around like I was a bloody
raw steak flopping onto the grill.

I was relieved to arrive in the recovery room. It was a
more intimate crowd now, just Connor, Claire, a nurse, and
me. It was a smaller room with dimmer lights. There were
blood stains on the floor. I wondered about the gory post-op
scenes these walls had witnessed and hoped I wouldn't be
one of them. I told myself to relax and breathe because the
worst was over, and finally, no one would be touching me,
inflicting violent pain for the first time in three days. It was
all over, I thought, and smiled watching Connor stand next
to my bed rocking Claire in his arms. She looked so tiny.
She had brown curly hair, matted with blood, but she
looked like the most beautiful creature to me.

The recovery nurse was a young and petite blonde with
a messy ponytail. She looked exhausted. I thought she
probably hadn't slept in a while, like us. She had clear
porcelain skin with dark purple eye circles. I couldn't
imagine how my own face looked. I was glad we all looked
like shit here.

The epidural quickly wore off. The pain was sharp and
intense at my incision. I felt it deep into my body in all 7
layers they'd severed and torn open. I struggled to breathe
because the movement of my diaphragm up and down was
too much on the incision. Even such a slight gentle

movement felt like it was tearing me in half. I was still so
dizzy and sleepy. I just wanted the pain to stop so I could
go to sleep.

Fundal Massage

"I'm really sorry, but I need to do a fundal massage
now. This will be uncomfortable," the nurse said.

Before I could internally translate that
"uncomfortable" is always code for painful around here,
she adjusted her feet into a power stance to muster all her
strength, balled her fists, and shoved her whole weight into
my sewn abdomen, digging and driving her elbows up and
down. My whole body reacted, folding upward as I
screamed in a deep voice like a cow mooing. This was yet
another threshold of pain I didn't think was possible for a
live human body.

"Oh God!" I screamed and gagged. I was genuinely
calling out to God to remove me from this body, to kill me.
I didn't recognize the tone from my own throat. It was
guttural. I hadn't ever heard that voice come out of me
before. This was a blinding, altering pain, and I looked at
the nurse in terror, too weak to lift my arms and fight her
off my body.

"Whoa what's going on? What are you doing to her?
She just had surgery!" Connor shot up from his plastic
folding chair, as he clutched Claire to his chest, thinking
the nurse must be killing me. He'd seen some shit through
this week, but never anything this violent.

Women in TikTok comment sections tried to warn me
of this technique, but I'd forgotten. It was one of the details
that fell through the cracks in my desperate studies. I tried
to remember every little detail of what to expect and what

would be expected of me, but it was impossible. Hundreds of women detailed the agony of the fundal massage.

"It was by far worse than labor," woman after woman yelled into the algorithm, hoping to reach the women to come after them, knowing that, once again, doctors or midwives never warn us of these experiences.

Surely, I thought, if you get a C-section, they'd never do this. Vigorously pressing and kneading directly into a deep and freshly sewn surgical wound could only be something you'd see in a gory horror film like Saw. But there she was, elbow deep in my abdomen as my eyes bulged and I held back vomit. Connor shushed Claire with tears in his eyes.

A fundal message is a technique performed on the uterus to stimulate contractions. It prevents postpartum hemorrhaging, according to the National Institutes of Health (NIH). I read that some hospitals do them as routine, whereas some do first a somewhat gentler fundal "check," to assess whether the full massage is necessary. A check is a similar maneuver, but less forceful. The nurse checks the firmness, position, and height of the uterus, or fundus. If it feels boggy and soft, a massage is required to coax the body to continue contracting to expel excess blood and tissue.

I whimpered as she stopped. I thought there was no way my stitches were still intact.

"I know. I'm so sorry. Unfortunately, I have to do that every 15 minutes for a while."

After the third massage, I begged her to stop. "I'm declining them. Please. I can't survive another one. I don't care if I die. I'd rather die," I said grabbing her hand. I tried to grip firmly so she'd take me seriously the way people do

in the corporate world during a handshake to establish
confidence, but I was so weak.

"I know. I'm so sorry," she said, looking at the clock
on the wall with a sigh.

"Everything has felt great down there so far, so I think
we might be safe to skip one," she whispered.

Holding her

"Do you want to hold your baby?" she asked me.
Baby? Hypnotized by the horror of this pain, I'd forgotten I
had one.

"We can try to sit you up just a little, enough to put her
on your chest," she offered. "She needs to eat. Let's try to
breastfeed her." I nodded, not able to speak. I couldn't
believe I'd have anything to offer this poor baby in the state
I was in. I felt no longer human, and yet she needed her
mother.

She placed this warm little creature on my chest, and I
tried my best to smile, but I had disassociated. My vision
was fuzzy from whatever meds they had running through
me. The nurse held her there in place, knowing I didn't
have the strength to be trusted to hold her on my own. I
wanted to be present for this monumental moment of
holding my baby for the first time, but I wasn't there. I
didn't know where I was or if I'd ever find myself again. I
don't know if I truly remember much of holding her or if I
am remembering a bit through the photo Connor took of us
the way we remember early childhood memories through
old home videos and stories our parents tell us. These
photos were a far cry from the pictures I'd imagined to star
in when I packed my makeup in my hospital bag and curled
my hair a few days ago. My eyes were still swollen, nearly

shut, and my skin was bright red from straining in pain for
hours.

I do remember that I looked down at my left breast as
the nurse placed Claire in front of it, guiding it to her
mouth.

"Wow, she latched right on there. That's impressive!"
she said with a smile.

"Oh, then we're doing it?" I asked. "Look, Connor!"

"Yeah girl! She's on there. Looks great," she said. I
was relieved that I'd finally done something right after
everything up until now had gone so horribly wrong and I
let my head fall back on the pillow until the next fundal
massage.

My next memory is in a different room on the
Postpartum Recovery floor. It was smaller than the L&D
room but still had a small bathroom with a shower and a
pleather bench that extended for Connor to sleep on. I had
tubes and wires coming out of every angle of my body. I
felt pressure on my legs and looked down to see that they'd
wrapped them from my ankles to my knees with warm
machines that sort of massaged me. I assumed they
prevented blood clots. All I wanted to do was sleep. I was
still piecing together where I was when I saw a new nurse
reading my chart on a wheeled computer machine of some
sort. All I could think about were the fundal massages.

"Can I please decline the fundal massages? I can't
handle that pain anymore," I said weakly to her.

"Not really honey," she said, keeping her eye contact
with the computer.

"Smell her head. She smells so good," Connor said,
smiling and holding Claire. He was having the magical
experience that I'd dreamed of having. He was in the

newborn bliss. Again, I'm reminded that there is a baby in the room.

The incision pain was intense. It burned and stung deeper than I'd ever felt. It reminded me of the horror movie *Ghost Ship.* There's a scene of people dancing in a ballroom when a thin, sharp wire flies through the crowd cutting everyone in half at the waist. I felt like I'd been through the same, cut in half irreparably. I thought if I took too deep of a breath or tried to adjust my position that my insides would spill out. It wasn't just the incision. I never had heard about how contractions continue after birth for sometimes days. Everyone knows contractions suck during labor, but somehow the lie has been that all the pain stops, and that it's nirvana as soon as the baby comes out. I breathed through each contraction until the sun came up.

32 Falling in Love

Claire would only sleep for about 10 minutes at a time, night or day. I was grateful to be awake for her every sound. I loved even her cry. She was crying for me, and I knew I was her comfort. I couldn't pick her up myself, but the nurse placed her gingerly in my arms for feedings. The cries stopped immediately as soon as we connected, reunited. It comforted me too to pull her close to my chest, like a relief I'd only feel when she was physically attached to me. My heart was living outside of my chest.

Connor had stopped at home for a few hours with the dogs again, and I was alone with my baby girl. The sun brightened the room, and I felt hope for the first time since I heard the word "C-section." Finally, I felt the warm fuzzies I'd felt robbed of overnight. She smiled peacefully in her sleep, and I stroked her dark brown hair. There she was. Her little face I'd ached to see and know inside me for almost the last year was now cupped into my palm. She smelled divine. The love I felt toward her was cosmic.

"I love you, Claire." I repeated softly, just above a whisper, rubbing my nose gently onto hers.

Over and over again, desperately, I'd tell her, but it never felt like enough. The word "love" didn't suffice. I loved my parents, loved Connor, loved Punkin, and loved my friends. I recognized "love," but this feeling was foreign and nothing of the sort. The fact that I had lived 30 years on earth and had this whole new range of emotion, that I'd never discovered before, intoxicated me. It was thrilling. I had no prior concept of this depth of human feeling. It was like I was only half-living before this. I'd now been cracked open with a nuclear explosion of warmth. This was so much more than love. It rather reminded me of the Greek word Agape, and I wished human vocabulary had the capacity to encapsulate such a phenomenon, whatever this force was between us. It made sense that it couldn't. This wasn't human, it was celestial. Agape has ancient origins and often describes the love between God and man. It's such a different love, incomparable, that humanity had to create another word for it. Otherworldly, that's what this was. Nothing and no one else mattered to me.

Connor felt his own version of it too. Before he left, he peered into her bassinet watching her sleep.

"I've never been this afraid to die before," he said.

"What do you mean?" I asked.

"I can't believe we have to one day leave her here on earth," he said with wet eyes.

I'd never leave her, I thought. Physical death couldn't separate me if, God forbid, anything happened to either of us, my soul would chase hers into death.

"Happy birthday, baby," I said to her.

We were indelibly one.

33 Postpartum Labor

The light shined through the window, and I knew it was daytime again. Connor stood up to stretch.

"My back hurts," he grunted. "They really should make these couches more comfortable." I didn't have the energy to point out how tone-deaf it was of him to complain to me about physical discomfort.

A midwife came into our room. She looked worried. She was one of many who saw me through my 3-day labor before her shift ended.

"I heard how everything played out," she said. "I'm so sorry."

She handed me a pamphlet titled, "Traumatic Birth." It recommended therapy services. It looked expensive. I still wasn't sure what the hospital bill would look like and didn't want more financial pressure. I was afraid to be honest with anyone about how I was really feeling. I was afraid they'd see me as a mentally unfit mother and take my baby from me. I wish I'd known how common my experience was. Why is this all a secret? After the books, the class, the appointments, the social media pages, the blogs… None of it had prepared me for the reality of birth.

I needed rest, but there was no time to sleep. I had to breastfeed Claire around the clock. My head bobbed as I fought for consciousness. I worried for my own physical health, but I felt like I wasn't allowed to think or ask about myself. I had just had serious major abdominal surgery. In any other healthcare situation, the patient would rest for weeks. As a new mother, the physical, mental, and emotional *labor* had just begun.

Connor leaned down over the clear plastic bassinet where Claire was sleeping. He was beaming and snapping pictures to send to our friends and family, all of whom were begging to come visit. I couldn't imagine seeing anyone.

"I'm going to let the dogs out again and hang out with them for a bit. I'll be back soon. I'll get us food. What do you want, sushi, wine?"

Throughout my pregnancy, I always told Connor I wanted a big gourmet sushi meal with a bottle of chilled Sancerre. I craved both the whole 10 months, and I couldn't wait to indulge in my favorites again. I'd hold my baby in one arm and chopsticks in the other hand.

Connor was tired, but chipper. He was excited and relieved that the hard stuff seemed to be over. Claire and I had both survived the birth, and the celebrations had begun. For him, the fun parts had started. He had no concept of how dire my state was. I couldn't believe he was leaving me alone with Claire for the fucking dogs for the hundredth time. I couldn't move from my supine position even the slightest. I couldn't stand or pick her up on her own, and he was leaving me alone with her. What if she needed me or started to cry? I still had a fucking catheter in for Christ's sake.

"I can't eat. I don't want anything. I feel so sick," I told him.

"You need to eat something. You haven't eaten anything but that gross beef broth since we got here last week." He was right. I thought I probably should give my body some sustenance.

"Can you order me a bagel?" I pointed to the menu on the side table with the hospital food options.

As much as I fought the sleep, I fell in and out of consciousness for most of the morning alone in the room with Claire, but I was startled awake sometimes as often as every five minutes with a knock on the door. Nurses, Nursing Assistants, Medical Assistants, Nursing Supervisors, Midwives, OBs, pediatricians, and medical students entered like a revolving door. A few times, multiple people came at the same time, and we had a line out the door. I wasn't even sure what they were doing to me. I was too tired to care. They'd take my blood pressure, give me pills to swallow, and ask if I'd passed gas yet. I was more concerned with Claire. In the haze, I tried hard to focus my eyes and stay alert as they pressed their stethoscopes on her little chest while she slept, swaddled in the plastic bassinet next to my bed. I was grateful when they'd pop in while I was breastfeeding so they could hold my head up and make sure I didn't fall asleep holding her.

I was startled again by the loud clicking of the door, but I exhaled with relief to finally see Connor again.

"How are my girls," he said with a smile, hands full of paper bags and to-go cups.

"Thank God it's you. What time is it?" I asked him, trying to sit up slightly because I kept sliding down in the slightly tilted bed.

"It's time to get that catheter out!" a nurse entered the room behind him, interrupting.

"Take it out? How will I pee? I can't move. I had a C-section," I informed her. She must have read my chart wrong, I thought. I hadn't moved a muscle yet. I looked to my left at the bathroom, which was about five feet from the bedside, but it may as well have been a mile. The catheter had been my favorite part of this whole process. By the end of the third trimester, I was peeing every 15 minutes, whether I was on a toilet or not. To not have to struggle my way to the bathroom was a luxury. She slid it out.

"Honey, it should only stay in there for about 24 hours, and we're already past that," she said. "Time to get you up and moving!"

She laughed at what must have been an incredulous expression on my face.

"We'll do it together! It's better for you to move early on. It helps you recover. The longer you lay there, the more painful it will be to get out of bed. Better to rip off the band-aid, so to speak!"

She bent below the bed pressing a button to slowly raise me from my horizontal position. I winced in pain as my weight shifted onto my incision, and I felt my organs fall into place. Everything felt loose in my torso like raw chicken breasts in a big plastic bag of sauce for marination.

I felt so nauseated and gagged at the bagel on the side table.

"That's normal. You might not have an appetite for a while. Your digestive system has been through a lot. Everything has to re-organize in there," she said.

Her phone clipped to her waistband rang, and I realized it's what happens when we press the call button on the bed.

"Let's start there. I'll be back, and we'll practice standing. Baby steps!" She reminded me of an older version of Luna Lovegood from Harry Potter. Her whimsical tone and positive attitude felt out of place. It felt like no one cared that I had just been through hell and back and had whiplash from the shock of each painful scene after another.

"Don't be a baby! You heard her you gotta move!" I turned my head toward Connor like the scene in The Exorcist. I didn't even have words, just silent rage with tears in my eyes as he joked.

Luna returned with her annoying pep in her step. "Time to stand!" I didn't return her smile.

She picked up one leg after another, slowly turning them like hands on a clock off to the left side of the bed as I winced. I could feel the parts of my incision, that had started to settle and heal in place, tear.

I took a deep breath sitting on the edge of the bed where she'd propped me up, feeling my feet touch the tile. I couldn't remember the last time I felt the floor.

She crouched down to my eye level. We held each other's focused gaze, gripping each other's forearms.

"On the count of three. It'll hurt, but push through."

I groaned and held onto her tightly. I was vertical. My organs sloshed around again, further down deeper into my body, and I felt more nauseous. Without asking, I started to lower back down in slow motion to the bed.

"Nice, babe!" Connor cheered me on from the couch eating a chicken tender.

"Take a moment, but we're going to walk," she said.

I'd have just ignored her, folded my arms and said like a child, "You can't make me!" But I had to pee, bad, and again I missed my catheter.

I looked to the bathroom, where I knew there would be the sweet relief of a toilet. I took a deep breath, linked forearms with Luna, and heaved myself into a vertical stance again. My legs felt like heavy immobile logs and my incision stung like hell, all the way deep into my center.

"I can't move," I said in a whiny tone, shaking my head. "You can," she corrected me. "You'll feel better once you pee!"

I looked down at my left foot as she adjusted a metal walker and shifted my weight from her arms to the handles. I shuffled a few inches forward. I never noticed before that

the lower abdominal muscles help us drive our legs forward
to walk. These were the abs the doctors had torn open with
their hands and sewn back together just hours ago. My legs
shook as I shuffled and groaned in pain with each mini
thrust forward. I finally made it to the toilet after probably
5 minutes.

"Now what?" I looked at Luna, feeling absolutely lost
at the thought of sitting down. This bitch was going to have
to pick me up and place me down there herself. I stood
there, frozen. She placed a higher toilet seat over top of the
toilet so it wouldn't be as far of a distance. I braced myself
on the cold metal bar on the wall, the other arm gripping
her. I got about half-way somehow leaning on everything
around me and started to pee. I stood there while she
changed my giant bloody pad and crepey paper shorts. As
much as I hated her for making me do this, I did feel a little
more human, relieved and fresh.

We'd repeat this every few hours, every time I had to
pee. I hated drinking water because I knew it meant another
trip. After a carton of grape juice, I was ready for Luna to
drag me over there again. We went through the same
routine. She got me all freshened up. About halfway off the
toilet, her phone rang.

"I gotta run! I'll be back to check on you," she said
hurrying out of the room. "I'm proud of you for how far
you've come today!"

Before I could say a word, my heart sank, realizing
that Connor was home with the damn dogs again. I was
alone. I was stuck. Claire was in that room, and I had to get
close to her. I took some breaths and heaved myself into a
slow shuffle across the room. I leaned back, slowly
swinging my right leg stiffly onto the bed. Half laying
down, my left leg was stuck hanging off the side along with

my left hip and half my weight. I usually needed Connor or Luna to pick up my left leg. I didn't have the abdominal strength or pain tolerance to lift it myself up and over the side of the mattress. I was stuck. Truly, I couldn't move. I tried. I looked around and saw my phone. I shimmied it into my fingers and pulled it into my hand. Holding my weight shakily with my palm, I stretched my fingers to put in my passcode and called Connor.

"Where are you," I asked him, crying.

"I just left the house, I'll be there in like 20 minutes," he said.

"Okay," I started to cry and hung up." Fuck. I couldn't stay here for 20 minutes, I thought. I looked around for my call button, my only hope. I had noticed the ones on the side of the bed didn't work by pressing them and getting no replies earlier in the week. The real one was on a remote with a thick wire attached to the electrical behemoth of a bed. I slid my hand, still holding my weight to the remote, carefully trying not to fall. I felt so guilty pressing the button. Nothing was wrong, I was just stuck. I felt pathetic as it rang.

"What's wrong?" a nurse's voice I didn't recognize answered with a ton of background noise. They were busy, and I felt even guiltier.

I was crying so much I couldn't speak clearly because they didn't understand me. I tried to say, "I'm stuck."

"She's crying," I heard her say to voices behind her more distantly. "We're on our way!"

The door burst open with three nurses. I felt like I was in trouble, like a child who'd gotten themselves into a situation of their fault and now needed to be rescued.

"Where is your baby," they said immediately, and I turned my head toward the bassinet. Claire was sleeping peacefully through this whole ordeal, swaddled in her little pink blanket and matching hat with a bow. I realized I scared them by crying they thought something was wrong with her.

"I'm sorry. I'm just stuck. I can't get my leg onto the bed," I cried. "I'm so sorry."

One scooped up my leg and the other caught my weight from my torso, relieving my shaking muscles.

"Don't apologize. That's what the button is for. We don't want you to hurt yourself," one of them said as she placed me back into my bed-prison.

The relationships between patients and nurses are so intimate. Though strangers, they care for us when we're at our most vulnerable. There are fantastic L&D nurses out there. I followed a few on TikTok, and they seemed like the only voices educating women on things that can go awry during labor.

34 Nightfall

Connor scooted the couch over to me so we'd feel closer together as if it was one big bed. Claire was at our feet in her plastic bassinet. He'd brought our blankets and pillows from home to give us some sense of comfort. The room looked like a slumber party as it darkened.

"Everyone's coming to visit tomorrow, so let's get some sleep." He pulled up our green floral comforter and rolled over to put his arm around me. We closed our eyes, and just as we relaxed, Claire cried.

"Will you hand her to me? Remember, I can't get her myself," I said sitting up, ready to clock in for my feeding shift.

He sighed and grunted, rubbing his eyes. He placed her in my arms and tucked himself back in. He fell asleep in seconds. I stared at her as she ate and nursed herself back to sleep. I typed the time in my phone so I wouldn't forget how long she fed and when she needed to eat next. The nurses had been asking me, and I learned my lesson to keep track.

"Connor!" I whispered aggressively to wake him up, yet quiet enough to not disturb Claire.

"What?" he startled awake.

"I need you to put her back in her bassinet, please," I gestured for him to take her.

He groaned. "I need to sleep."

I refrained from saying, "How do you think I feel fuckface?" I closed my eyes instead. I fell into something that wasn't quite sleep, more of a twilight, knowing the quiet would only last for a short time.

Ten minutes later, she cried, startling us both awake. After the fourth waking, Connor was panicked.

"Oh my God. Call the nurse. She needs to go to the nursery, please. I need to fucking sleep," Connor huffed and puffed out of the couch-bed.

"This is what it's like to have a baby," I said slowly to try to calm him and her at the same time.

When she was done eating, I did call. I didn't want her away from me, but I figured I'd be a better and safer parent if I got some sleep. It had been so many days I didn't remember the last time I slept more than a few minutes. I worried Connor had no idea what he was in for. He hadn't read the books and flooded his algorithms with educational baby parenting content. I knew then that I was about to tackle the fourth trimester somewhat alone. I didn't want to separate from Claire, but this night with the nursery would be my last reprieve and only shot at sleep.

"Hi, can I please send Claire to the nursery for just a bit so I can sleep?" I said into the remote.

"Sure. I'll be right there." It was a new nurse for the night shift. I saw the name Lexi written on the whiteboard on the wall with a smiley face. I liked her because I didn't have to beg her for my pain meds. They gave me Tylenol and Oxy, but I had to ask at least twice to get the Oxys. I guessed they were worried about addiction. I felt gross and misunderstood needing them so badly. I was still in so much pain. When I'd asked the nurses when the pain would stop, they told me it gets better after two weeks.

"I'll bring her back when she needs to eat," Lexi said softly. "Hi baby," she said to Claire as she walked out the door. She seemed nurturing, and I trusted her.

I blinked and she was back. I looked at the clock on the wall and noticed it had been an hour. I felt refreshed, somehow. Connor was still asleep. I didn't care to wake him. I was so happy to see Claire. I reached for her. "My girl," I said in a motherly tone that confirmed the role for me. I sounded like a loving mom. If nothing else, the love came naturally to me.

35 Intruders

"My parents are on their way. When's your family coming?" he asked me, as if I seemed ready for company. I looked down at my blood-filled diaper and completely exposed chest.

"I mean the nurses are in here every 15 minutes to perform new sadistic acts of torture on my naked body, so I'm not really in a rush, Connor," I said. In cinematic timing, a new nurse appeared.

She had a pin of *Mrs. Doubtfire* with a little quote that said, "Help is on the way dear!" It was one of my favorite movies. I'd dressed up as Mrs. Doubtfire for Halloween once, and I immediately liked her. I watched her write "Emily" on the white-board.

Emily pulled the covers off me and unwrapped me layer by layer to examine my incision. She pulled my paper undies down to assess how much blood was in there. Connor's parents would walk in the door any minute, and I was ass-naked and bloody.

I was relieved when she walked out, but before the door shut, his parents walked in.

All my research had recommended no visitors at all until after 4 weeks, given newborns' lack of immune system. The secret threads of TikTok comments all warned me that, even if it were my wishes to have no visitors, they'd show up anyway. Everyone is excited to meet the baby. There were safer ways to do it. Some hospitals, if they allow visitors at all, only allow them for 15 minutes at a time, making room for the revolving door of grandparents, siblings, and close friends.

This baby was part of my body since the dawn of her existence until less than 24 hours ago. Now, I had to watch as my most precious organ sat in someone else's arms, away from me. I felt helpless like I had no control to protect her.

"Where is she?" they said, beaming. I couldn't blame them for their enthusiasm. They were excited to see their first grandchild. I faked a smile and pulled a sheet over my chest.

"Just no kissing her, please," Connor said, hoping they could hear over their blinding joy.

I remembered my long-time client Clint's warning to me months prior. "Don't let anyone touch her, Katie." I knew that he had recently lost a child. I didn't dare ask for details, but when I was in my third trimester, he shared more. He and his wife had relatives over to meet the new baby. Someone kissed him, and he got RSV, a deadly respiratory virus commonly passed to babies from relatives kissing them. He died in the hospital a week later. I'd seen similar stories all over TikTok, warning me of the same.

I watched Connor's mom, hold Claire to her chest on the couch Connor had reconstructed.

"She's beautiful!" she said.

I could smell her perfume and Connor's dad's cologne or after-shave from across the room. I'd learned that fragrance was detrimental to newborns. Bonding and feeding are driven by hormones, which are driven by scent. The mother needs to smell the baby's pheromones and the baby needs to smell the mother's. I stunk to high heaven. Apparently, the body expels intense bodily odor from the armpits to help the baby identify the mother and feed. When people wear fragrances, it can negatively affect milk supply and throw these necessary hormones off balance.

These chemicals are also irritants to their delicate skin and respiratory systems, which is why you can't even use normal laundry detergent to wash their clothes. There she was, drenched in a storm of thick fragrance. The nurses would notice later, and they bathed her in the sink.

Before I gave birth, I had a shared list with Connor with a pre-scripted text message to send to our friends and family detailing our wishes. It read:

"Hi family and friends, Katie and Claire are resting, and we appreciate your patience. We'll let you know when we're ready for visitors. For those coming to the hospital, we have a few asks:

- Please no heavy perfume or cologne. Fragrance can be dangerous for newborns.

- Please do not kiss her. We understand you want to express your love. Her little body doesn't have an immune system and RSV is going around.

- Please only stay for 15min at a time each.

- Skin-to-skin contact for mom is very important and you may not get to hold her for as long as you'd like

Thanks for understanding!"

In all the madness, I forgot to remind him. This is another benefit of having a doula. They remember things like this in the postpartum blur and help coach the new dads too. I didn't remember it until I was tilted on my side while the nurses examined my asshole in front of everyone, a moment of true humility.

I tried to participate in small talk when nurse Emily reappeared. "I see we have visitors! I'll try to be quick."

She undressed me below the waist as Connor held a blanket to shield his parents' eyes from my bloody genitals. She changed my bandages and examined me. The room smelled like lochia. I learned the flow postpartum has an earthy and metallic smell, like a swamp. This felt like another private moment, and I couldn't believe people other than the nurse were in the room, just a few feet from the bed. I was humiliated.

An hour passed. "I have to feed her again" I said to Connor, gesturing to hand Claire back to me.

I thought that they'd take the social cue that I was about to take my breast out, and it would be time to give me some privacy. They stayed, too enamored with the baby. I handed Connor a blanket to shield me again, as I struggled to get Claire to latch. The fragrance scents all over her burned the back of my throat. My sense of smell was stronger than ever, even stronger than it had been during pregnancy.

"God, I can't get it. I need the nurse," I told Connor in a frustrated tone, trying to get his attention while he socialized. I felt anxious because I knew his parents were waiting for me to be done feeding her so they could have her back. In serendipitous timing, the door clicked open, and Emily appeared.

"Can you help me get her to latch?" I looked down, unsure what I was even looking for. All I knew was that breastfeeding hurt like a bitch. The nurse adjusted Claire's lips. She noticed my grimace, trying to conceal my pain to not make our guests feel uncomfortable.

"Breathe through the first 15 seconds. Then, you're in the clear." She was right. It hurt like it was a fat blade sliding out of me instead of milk.

Another hour passed. "Connor, can you help me to the bathroom?" I asked, embarrassed and interrupting their family bliss.

I groaned and cried as Connor and Emily peeled my body parts off the bed, and I gripped the walker and shuffled slowly again to the bathroom. We barely fit in the room and struggled to close the door so his parents couldn't see me naked on the toilet.

"I'm sorry, but it's time for your parents to go," I mouthed silently to him, eyes wide, as I held onto his arms for balance. He nodded and lowered me onto the toilet.

"I know," he mouthed back.

I was sweating and out of breath. He picked me up off the toilet and changed the bloodied diaper, gently wiping me. I didn't even fart in front of Connor and always tried to keep the gross parts of me private. I felt completely vulnerable and wondered if he'd still be attracted to me after all of this. I shuffled back to the bed, unable to politely hide my pain. I struggled my way onto the bed, Connor lifting my legs and tucking me in as I cried.

"Okay guys, it's time to go. They need to rest," Connor said with a sweeping motion pointed toward the door.

"When can we come back tomorrow?" they asked. "I don't know. We'll text you," he said.

A team of nurses appeared, and Connor threw his head back, realizing we wouldn't get a moment alone. Carly and Leah stopped by next, but I don't even remember them being there. I only believe it because there's a photo of Carly next to the hospital bed with a swollen whale-like creature holding Claire, whom I assume to be me.

My dad and Sandy agreed to come the following day. Per Luna's advice, I shuffled to the shower to practice standing and washed myself. "It'll help you feel more like you," she said.

I applied some makeup, wanting to look as decent as possible for my dad. I didn't want him to worry about me. I sat up in bed, ready to be spritely.

Connor's parents were excited to spend more time with Claire and came again, so rather than alone time with my dad, it became the first meeting of the in-laws. They all ooed and awed over the baby and small talked while I wondered if anyone remembered I was there.

"How are you feeling?" my dad asked me. Finally, someone saw me and not just the baby. I knew she was the star of the show here, rightfully so, but I'd just been through so much. I wanted someone to care.

"I feel good. I'm sore, but I'm just so excited that she's finally here!" It was only a half-lie. I was over the moon in love with her, but I downplayed the pain, as most women do. After a hello-hug, he stood at the foot of my bed and stayed there with his hands behind his back and admired Claire from across the room while Sandy held her, taking turns with Connor's mom. He hated hospitals and was a huge germaphobe. He always carried a little plastic device to avoid pressing buttons on public elevators and kept hand sanitizer on him at all times. On his birthdays, he'd wave a paper plate to extinguish the candle flames rather than blow on the candle and spray germs on the cake. I knew this was his worst nightmare to come here and be under the same roof as sick people, and it meant a lot to me that he came. Seeing him reminded me of who I was. I remembered that I was a person, even if she was still a stranger.

36 Eviction

"Once you prove you can walk and we get your pain more under control, you're going home," Luna woke me up and told me. "I requested a physical therapist for you, and no more of this!" She folded up the walker and took it out of the room. I felt like she'd left me out at sea without a raft.

Home? I'd forgotten I even had one. I had been in the hospital for a week. Connor only got five days off work for the birth. He didn't qualify for paternity leave at his job until he'd been there for a year, and it had only been 6 months. The time they gave him was already a favor they did off the record. Like its lack of generosity with maternity leave, the US offers no paid paternity leave either. Some companies in recent years have begun to offer a few days or a few weeks for dads. In most other countries, like Japan, fathers get up to a year of paid leave. We assumed we'd spend 2 days in the hospital and rest at home caring for the baby for the rest. Now his clock had run out, but we weren't even out of the hospital yet. I was about to be home alone, bedridden and unable to even wipe my own ass.

Is it safe to go home?

I wasn't just afraid I'd be stuck in bed. I was scared for my safety. According to the NIH, US prenatal and postpartum care guidelines had last been updated in 1930. What the fuck? With all the modern technological and medical advancements, how could women be so left behind? If the nurses were coming in every 5 minutes at the hospital to check my vitals and see if I was about to have a stroke from preeclampsia or bleed out from hemorrhaging, how could I just go home and hope for the best?

Among pregnancy related deaths, 53% occur postpartum, according to a CDC article about Maternal Mortality, studying cases across 2017-2019. I'd read the stats and didn't want to be a part of them. I thought back to videos I'd seen from other countries of luxurious and comforting postpartum centers. Some cities in the US have them too, but they're only for the rich. Women would stay in a hotel-like environment with a full nursing staff helping them around the clock for physical therapy, lactation consulting, and overall baby-training. Each meal was catered to postpartum nutrition and delivered like room service. I thought of the book, *Bringing Up Bebe,* and how the author, an ex-pat who gave birth in France, described her longer hospital stay after birth. Even without a C-section, she got five days of recovery in the hospital. I was angry that the US healthcare system discarded postpartum women so carelessly despite the research proving danger.

"When will I come back to get checked out?" I asked the team of doctors and nurses, one of the many groups coming in and out.

"On the second day of being home, you'll go to the pediatrician's office to make sure she's gaining weight," the OBGYN said, nodding. "Make sure dad can come with you because you can't lift more than 10 pounds, and your baby is 8 pounds. Don't try to lift the car seat."

Connor rubbed his hand over his brow. "All right. I'll talk to my boss and see if they'll give me off work for a few hours again." He was stressed about making a bad impression with his new company.

I felt guilty, but I didn't have anyone else. Everyone in our life also worked fulltime or lived out of town. Had I known we'd be here this long, I'd have planned better postpartum help. I was so worried about the birth that I'd forgotten the hard part would begin after it. I couldn't believe I'd have to leave home and make it to an appointment in this state. I couldn't imagine even being in a car. I'd searched online and found that other countries send a medical professional to the woman's home, rather than making her leave the house mid-recovery.

"Okay, I'll call and make that appointment today for her, but what about me? When do I get checked out?" I asked meekly.

"You'll have your post-op appointment here at two weeks and then your six-week appointment to clear you for activity and make sure you're healing well," she said looking up from her clipboard. "Actually, you should call today so you can get in. It's tough."

Two weeks. I just had to survive two weeks before I'd have the mental relief of knowing I was okay, that my stitches were still intact and my organs weren't going to fall out. I remembered hearing about postpartum preeclampsia and tried to remember where I put my at-home blood pressure cuff. My survival and Claire's survival were in my hands for the next two weeks, and I was ready to play doctor and single mom while Connor was at work.

Postpartum Care

I called the midwives office desk to schedule those two- and six-week appointments, barely able to see the numbers I dialed through the brain fog of the painkillers and sleep deprivation.

"Hmm…" The office receptionist clicked through the calendar. "I'm trying to find a spot for you, but it looks like we're full in every location. This is our busy season. Everyone's having babies this time of year."

"Full? I'll come early in the morning or evening or something… Please. What do I do if there's no appointment? Where else can I go?"

This wasn't a hair appointment to get my roots touched up, this was my life and physical health. We'd pre-booked all third trimester appointments to ensure I could get in at the right times but there was nothing planned for *after* the baby came out. I felt I no longer mattered.

"Let me talk to the midwives and see if there are any appointments we can move around. We'll do our best, and I'll call you back," she said slowly, sensing the panic in my voice. She never called back. I called every few days to see if there had been any cancellations or other offices I could go to. I never got my two-week appointment and felt lucky to be healthy and alive. I did get a 6-week appointment scheduled for my 7th week. It felt like I'd landed a reservation at an exclusive restaurant like The Polo Bar in New York.

Graduating the Hospital

Next up on the revolving door of our hospital room was the Physical Therapist. "Hi, I'm Nicole! I'm here to help you learn to walk so you can go home."

My head bobbed as I mustered a reply. "Hi." I didn't have it in me for pleasantries. The painkillers made me so drowsy I wondered if she was a dream.

"Did they give you the wrap to go around your waist? The pressure holds everything in place as you move around, and it really helps with the pain and healing," she said.

I pulled up my gown and we looked down at my belly, wrapped in layers like a mummy (no pun intended). First, my giant diaper-pad soaked in blood, the crepey paper shorts, a lidocaine patch, an ice pack, and a thick white stretchy wrap to hold it all in place. That must be it, I thought.

"Wear that as much as you can while you're moving. How many stairs do you have at home?"

"A lot. I'm so scared. I have like 15 steps to get into our house from the outside and then I'll need to go up and down 15 more inside in between my bedroom and the bathroom," I whined. "Should I just get a hotel room for a week?"

"Hold a pillow like this on your belly, and do the stairs sideways like this," she held a pillow to her lower body and held out the other arm in front of her gripping an imaginary railing and inching her feet to the side.

She peeled me out of bed and returned my precious walker Luna had hidden from me. I squinted at the lights in the hall. I hadn't left this room in so long I didn't realize how dark it was in there. She pointed to a painting on the wall about halfway down the hallway.

"Let's make it to that picture. Go as slow as you need. If you can make it there, you can make it home," she said like a soccer coach with a pep talk before a big game.

Little did she know I sucked at sports too.

I stared at the painting as a focal point and drove one foot after another for each shuffling motion, clicking and clacking the walker in front of me. "I'm doing it!" I huffed.

"I know!" She laughed. "Let's ditch this walker. You can do it." I felt frozen as she took it away. She held me in a standing position while I got my bearings, and after a minute, I let go. It was like riding a bike for the first time when my dad let go of me, training wheels off, letting me peddle through the asphalt parking lot. My legs felt like they didn't belong to me.

"Let's go, babe!" Connor peaked his head out of the room with Claire in his arms. He looked down at her, "Go Mummy!"

I touched the painting and reluctantly declared, "I'm going home."

37 Home

Claire and I both had "going home outfits," but I didn't care anymore what we looked like and laughed at the idea. I just wanted to take refuge in the familiar soft bed and comfort of our bedroom. Connor helped me step into the foot holes of my soft gray stretchy pants and pulled them up over my still distended belly. The thought of being home, tucked in with Claire with no staff interrupting our bonding gave me the bravery to embark on the upcoming car ride. I'd cleaned the house like a nesting mad women the two weeks leading up to the birth. In some physical feat, I scrubbed the base boards, dusted the bookshelves, cleaned and re-organized all the dishes and pots and pans, and vacuumed the layers of dog hair that accumulated quickly on the floors after a few hours. I was excited to feel clean at home, away from the germs, blood stains, and pee-smell of the hospital.

A patient escort helped me sit into a big wheelchair and rolled me down the hall. Connor followed behind him wheeling a sleeping Claire and our bags on a cart. We landed in the lobby and headed toward the big revolving door as the self-playing piano played Beethoven's Fur Elise. The door spun and the warm summery outside air felt foreign in my lungs. I hadn't been outside in a week. I hadn't seen the sunlight or breathed fresh air in so long I felt like I was a space explorer who'd just landed on an alien planet, apprehensive about this mysterious atmosphere.

"I can't believe I have to go back to work tomorrow," Connor said as his Sunday scaries began to kick in with the sunset above the traffic. "I'm sorry."

"Maybe they'll let you out early," I said gripping the handle above my head and breathing through the sting of each pothole as they shook loose my recovering guts.

I looked up at the steps to the house like a Hobbit staring up at Mount Doom in *The Lord of The Rings*. I remembered the Physical Therapists advice to hold my pillow to my abdomen and mimicked her demonstration, gripping the railing and pulling myself sideways while Connor and Claire waited at the top.

The dogs were jumping and barking, riling up the rest of the neighborhood dogs. I knew we couldn't go in there. The cacophony startled Claire awake, and she cried. "Go in there and lock them in the fucking office," I snapped. "They're going to damage her ear drums! Her hearing is delicate!"

Finally, I made it into the house. The dogs were still barking, excited to see us after a week away, and the office door rumbled as they tried to barge through it. I looked around, and the house I'd left pristinely tidy was a mess. Connor had been there in and out all week and trashed it. I could tell that every time he had been there, he was in a rush to get in and out. I realized then how much and how often I cleaned up after him and the dogs. Without me here to do so, there was a carpet-like layer of dog hair on every surface of the house, muddy pawprints on everything, dishes in the sink, laundry all over the dining room table, and crumpled paper towels on the counters.

"How did you manage to ruin this house like this? I can't even clean now," I said on the verge of tears. I headed directly for the stairs to get up to my bedroom and get

Claire away from the filth and noise. This was far from the vision of bringing my baby home for the first time I'd always imagined, calm, quiet, clean, and sweet.

I felt like I'd boarded a ship destined for an iceberg. I was out to sea, and we were sinking.

38 Postpartum Animal Aversion

I know it sounds weird, but it's a real condition. I'd never heard of it either, until I got it myself. A mother becomes a creature non-mothers can never understand. I no longer related to non-mothering women. They felt like a different species to me. I used to be one of them, but I was now absolutely something else. I'd heard of women rehoming their dogs after having a baby and clutched my pearls at the unimaginable cruelty. I could have never understood. My own parents gave away their dog, Chancey, when I was a baby. He was a black mut with a white scruffy chin. My mom adopted him as a rescue and lived as his loving dog-mom for years. My mother adored animals. We were constantly at animal sanctuaries with a rescued bird in a shoebox she'd found on the road or an orphaned bunny. Her compassion toward all living things was unmatched, and I knew for her to let go of an animal she *loved,* the situation must have been dire. When she and my dad brought me home from the hospital, Chancey drooled and growled licking his lips and chomping to get a bite of my tiny body. He had to go, they decided. Connor's friends had a rescue dog, Boo, they loved deeply as their "daughter" but rehomed after having a baby too. Another friend from grade school had two large doodle dogs, and when she had her first baby, the dogs never came back into that house. I couldn't believe people could be so heartless, until I became a mother.

"Keep those dogs away from the baby, honey. Remember that news story a while ago where the girl put her baby's car seat down…and…" Sandy, a dog lover, said covering her face and shaking her head at the unspeakable.

I knew what local tragedy she was referring to. In fact, I'd heard multiple stories where parents brought home their babies, and the once gentle family pet ate the baby or bit their face, permanently disfiguring them.

From the moment we conceived, I was on guard, afraid one of them would step on my belly or jump at me with forceful paws, accidentally ending this little miracle growing inside me. I typically had bruises all over my body from them pawing me or knocking me over, but now my body was delicately creating life. I was scared every time I walked in the door and Punkin jumped for joy at my waist as I reminded him, "Sit!"

Connor saw gentle giants. I began to see giant threats. Still, I loved them, especially Punkin, while I was still pregnant. I felt guilty that our relationship had changed and that I looked at him now with fear instead of love. The night before my induction, I struggled down to the floor and let Punkin sit close to me. He placed his paw into my palm, and I stroked it like always.

"You'll always be my baby too. Things will be different, but don't worry," I smiled at him and kissed his head.

When I returned from the hospital, raw and bloodied with my guts freshly stitched shut, I desperately needed a tranquil postpartum oasis of quiet and clean. As I walked into the front door, I held Claire's ears shut tightly as she looked up at me, scared. The downstairs office door rumbled and boomed like thunder as they both barked and threw their 200 pounds of body against it. They'd missed me, but their excitement could so easily kill her or me in this fragile state. The rest of the neighborhood dogs had now chimed in too. I was so worried about her delicate eardrums. I may as well have run a jackhammer next to her head. I knew newborns needed quiet environments, and I felt like a failure for not providing one. I clutched her in my left arm close to my heart, cupping her ears. I walked sideways up the stairs wincing in pain as Connor yelled and scrambled through the office door to try to extinguish the chaos.

I looked down at my feet. They were covered in a thick layer of dog hair and dust. I usually vacuumed and broomed the floors twice daily just to keep it at bay. Without me here for a week, canine filth had taken over my home. It smelled like Taz. No matter how many baths he got, he could stink up a blanket or room in minutes. It took hours of cleaning to keep up, and I no longer had the hours to give.

When I reached refuge in my bed, my incision was on fire and bleeding a little. I'd walked too fast to escape from the noise. They were still barking, and Connor was yelling at them now, completely overwhelmed. I heard the office door swing open hard and slam into the wall, denting the drywall. They stampeded through the house as Connor wrangled them toward the backyard to blow off all this steam. I needed him here with me to cater to *our* needs while I was bedbound, but he needed to deal with them, and it was nearly a full-time job. I missed the hospital. It was the last place I felt some semblance of rest. I realized then that, with dogs, I'd be getting none here.

I stayed awake with Claire all night, again and again, unsure of the passage of days. She cried in my arms in between cluster feeding around the clock. I rocked her in the dark, smiling at her crying face, just happy to be with her in delirious elation. Connor had work in the morning and slept peacefully undisturbed on the couch downstairs. The solitude reminded me his life would not change much, while mine was entirely no more, replaced by my new identity as a mother.

Connor left for work early in the mornings, and we were alone all day, usually hiding in the bedroom from the predators awaiting us downstairs. Around noon, for the first time in three days, Claire drifted to sleep in my arms. I desperately tried to take advantage, not knowing how many minutes I'd have left before she wanted to latch again. I gently placed her slowly in her bassinet next to me, my healing abs splitting and stinging with the movement. Softly, she hit the miniature mattress. I laid myself back sighing into the soft pillows. I closed my eyes and immediately drifted. It was my first taste of sleep in more than 10 days.

Seconds later I gasped with my heart pounding and eyes wide open. Claire and I were both startled frantically out of our precious sleep that had taken days to achieve. Taz was walking around and panting downstairs. The sound of his toenails clicking loudly on the hardwood as he dragged his heavy paws with each step echoed up the staircase and through the door. Punkin followed him around, toenails just as loud, panting, grunting, and snorting. They weren't even doing anything wrong. This was just how loud they naturally were. Claire's loud crying had just stopped for the first time in so long. I had finally heard nothing but the ringing left in my ears from the aural overload, and the dogs ripped the moment out of my hands. We were so tired. Sleep was the only place I could escape the pain and my eyes were heavy. This was a postpartum torture chamber. I was overstimulated in a state of complete sensory overload at all times. Constant noise.

Another night passed without me noticing, only realizing the earth had spun by the sun shining through my bedroom window. It was dawn now, but days and nights were exactly the same. There was no difference in routine. Morning, noon, night, dawn, I breastfed Claire without sleep or food. I didn't remember if Connor had come home yet. If he did, I didn't notice.

Every night from 8-10pm, deep into the newborn witching hour, Connor put the dogs in the office with him to get them away from us while he played video games with them at his side. I suffered alone through more sleepless nights. I imagined if we didn't have the dogs, Connor would hold and rock Claire while I napped. With him being the only one here to care for them, Claire and I came last on the list. He fed them, bathed them, clipped their toenails, brushed them, and walked them. All while I breastfed, changed diapers, rocked and shushed, and bathed Claire. I developed her brain with black and white cards with shapes. I sang songs and read books. I massaged her with baby lotion. I tracked inventory and stocked her diapers and supplies. I dressed her and kept her clothes organized while I only changed my own clothes twice a week. I scheduled her doctor's appointments and followed the pediatrician's instructions carefully. We'd become separate single parents, I of Claire, and he of the dogs. Even when Connor took them away for a while in the evenings, our neighbors' dog next-door barked incessantly below our window. They'd gotten multiple citations from the city already from other neighbors complaining about the noise, and I knew there wasn't anything we could do to stop it.

Getting some fresh air

After two weeks, when I could walk comfortably for short distances, I decided we'd go outside for some peace and quiet, finally escaping the dogs. I felt so depressed and heavy, and I figured sunshine might help.

I remembered Nietzsche once said, "Never trust a thought that occurs to you indoors."

The pediatrician told us that sunlight is vital for newborns for both vitamin D and to establish their circadian rhythm, which teaches them to sleep at night and be awake during the day. I packed her into her stroller and grunted my way through lifting and piecing together the parts, just as Connor taught me. I stood back with my hands on my hips and smiled at my sculpture, my engineering feat. We walked around the block. The vibration of the sidewalk and her first taste of quiet without dogs sent her immediately to sleep. Since I hadn't seen her truly sleep before, I panicked for a moment and checked for her breathing. Her chest rose up and down, just as it should. Her face fell into relief like she could finally relax, and so could I. I wondered if I'd fall asleep while walking. I wished I could fit in the stroller to sleep next to her right there on the sidewalk. My nervous system felt calm, and my heartbeat slowed for the first time in two weeks. Suddenly, the tall plastic fence in the yard next to us thundered and shook forward with a loud barking inches from us. Claire's eyes shot open with a terrified facial expression, followed by the familiar sound of her crying. The sound we'd be retreating from at home was closer and louder than ever. I clutched Claire's ears and worried they'd be damaged for good this time. I hobbled the stroller forward with my waist, the handle painfully stretching my incision and tearing at the scabbing progress it had made. "Fucking dogs," I said out loud. I fucking hated them and felt a burning violent rage toward any animal that crossed my path like a mother bear with her cub, ready to kill anything threatening her. I imagined running over the birds and squirrels with the stroller's wheels and my face was hot with rage. We both cried the whole way home, back to our loud house with toenails and English bulldog noises. "It's okay baby I'm sorry," I said over the noise. I looked around the living room and dining room.

"You gotta be fucking kidding me," I said into the void. Taz had thrown up all over the floor. At 150 pounds, he pukes gallons. I couldn't crouch, squat, and bend down for the hours of cleaning this mess required.

"You have to come home and deal with them. Your dog threw up everywhere," I texted Connor, resenting him for even bringing them into my life and ruining my precious house.

For months, I'd try to read books to Claire at home. Reading to babies is good for their brain, according to my pregnancy studies. Unless Connor was home to take the dogs outside, I couldn't read to her at home. I couldn't read in a yelling tone to this newborn baby, "GOODNIGHT MOON" in her face. The dogs were ruining my ability to be a good mother, I thought.

One day, I'd finally made it to the couch and reclaimed my living room. I hadn't sat on the couch in months, sequestered to the bed upstairs. Claire had on a soft pink onesie. She looked so pure, a little pink angel from Heaven. Taz was snoring on the new bed on the floor we'd bought them that only lasted 3 weeks. It took up most of the living room. I ignored them and sang, "My Girl," to Claire.

Midway through the first verse something crawled across her torso. I shot up into action. It was a tick. It had made its way from the dogs, probably onto the couch, and now onto my delicate baby girl. At the same moment, the back door slammed open, and I heard Punkin's snorting and gargling. He galloped into the living room and unknowingly wiped his ass all over the beige couch. There was dog poop smeared everywhere and muddy pawprints all over the hardwood. Before I could deal with the mess, I grabbed a t-shirt next to me and snatched the tick off Claire's chest just before it touched her skin. Was she seconds away from Lyme Disease, I worried. We had tick medicine for the dogs. It's great for them because it prevents the ticks from latching onto their skin, but it meant they'd jump or fall off elsewhere. One time, before I was pregnant, Connor was laying shirtless next to me in bed. When I woke up, I rolled over to cuddle under his arm before I noticed a tick with its head burrowed deep into his flesh, legs hanging out behind it. Now one had reached my baby, risking her health and safety yet again.

"I do not want the dogs anymore. We need to re-home them. I do not want to live with them anymore," I stated to Connor like it was a legal statement. "Dogs do NOT belong in a home with a baby."

"Oh stop. They love you," he said, brushing me off. We were yelling over the noise of them walking around the kitchen.

"I don't fucking love them," My serious tone had crumbled. "I fucking hate them. They need to leave. I can't wait for them to die," I cried and slammed a bottle down on the counter, covering my face. It was so cruel, I know, but I couldn't help it. My animal instinct to protect my baby overtook compassion for any other species.

My phone must have been listening because, during my overnight scrolling with Claire in my arms, a video popped onto my FYP from a new mom. She was crying to other moms, in our very secret club of motherhood, about how she felt crazy for suddenly hating her once beloved dog. I opened the comments and thousands of women discussed "Postpartum Animal Aversion" or "Postpartum Pet Aversion." It's not only a natural reaction to the overstimulation and germs, but it's actually a very common hormonal response. It's a condition women usually keep to themselves. I could see why. These moms were met with comments of non-mothers who, like the old me, thought these women were evil sociopaths.

"This intense judgment toward women experiencing something very real, and a literal hormonal condition, is exactly why women don't talk about the real postpartum shit," one commenter wrote. "Look how many thousands of women agreed and were brave enough to admit it, and look how you're treating them!"

The dogs stayed in our lives, much to my chagrin. We didn't have the heart to send them to another family. The animal aversion stuck around and started to taper off when Claire was about a year old.

I'm not urging you to get rid of your dogs. I'm telling you this so that, if you have pets, you and your household can *prepare* for how things may need to change in your home to make room for a baby. This is all about empowering you with knowledge so that you're ready.

39 Breastfeeding

Becoming my baby's food source was a major undertaking no doctor, nurse, friend, or family member truly prepared me for. In fact, nobody brought up breastfeeding at all, other than how amazing it is. I'd been so focused on birth that I hadn't researched it much until I was already *in* it. Firstly, I was surprised to learn that it freaking hurts, at least at first. In the early days, when she'd latch, a pain stabbed all the way through my milk ducts and nipple until about 15 seconds of feeding. I clutched my sheets and breathed through it as it waned. After that, it felt like a release, and after those first few days, it became all I wanted to do. It was hard, but I loved it.

It's a completely full-time job, and women don't get enough credit for the commitment and toll it takes on the body. It's estimated that a woman will spend at least 1,800 hours or more breastfeeding in one year. Breastfeeding uses the same metabolic energy as walking seven miles in a day, taking 25% of the mother's caloric needs. It's also understood that these energy levels are probably even higher in the early days after birth.

Breastmilk is a fascinating liquid gold. It changes its nutritional value daily, tailored to the baby's current needs and developmental stage. For example, it even increases in water content during hot weather, according to the Western Missouri Medical Center website. The breasts also detect the baby's body temperature and regulate it for them.

Breastmilk also serves as the baby's immune system for the first 6 months. Women have an instinct to kiss their babies often. It's not only out of love. It's an information gathering system. As they kiss their skin, moms' brains send the recipe needed to create antibodies tailored to the baby's needs to fight off bacteria and viruses. I thought again of how cruel it is that American babies are torn from their working mothers' breasts.

When we'd go at the pediatrician for a cold, cough, or fever they'd say, "There is no treatment for viruses except time and breastfeeding."

Breastfeeding research suggests that it lowers risk for a myriad of diseases or illnesses for the baby including Sudden Infant Death Syndrome (SIDS), Type 2 Diabetes, Leukemia, Celiac, Asthma, and Bacterial Meningitis.

Benefits for Mom

Milk is made from the mother's blood, and creating it depletes her of vitamins and minerals. Careful nutrition and rest are essential. Although draining, when given the right support, it benefits mom too. Breastfeeding has been shown to lead to quicker recovery, and a lowered risk for postpartum depression. Nursing sends signals to the uterus to contract after birth and ease the body back to its pre-pregnancy state. It also helps the mother to prevent cancer.

According to the NIH, "Several large studies have shown extended lactation is associated with reduced risk of premenopausal breast, ovarian and endometrial cancers."

The research also suggests it protects women from other health conditions like osteoporosis, Type 2 Diabetes, high blood pressure, and cardiovascular disease.

According to the Cleveland Clinic, research has shown that the unique bonding experience breastfeeding offers may help reduce social and behavioral problems in both children and adults.

I personally loved the convenience of it. I didn't have to spend the precious minutes in between feeds frantically washing and sanitizing bottles, I never had to go to the kitchen throughout the night to make a bottle, and I never had to worry when we left the house if I'd forgotten anything. Once I'd gotten the hang of it, all I had to do was lift my shirt.

Breastfeeding in the US

Despite the benefits, American women breastfeed far less than anywhere else in the world. Women feel pressure to get back to work and stop breastfeeding after a few months, if at all, which is great for the American formula corporations. I read numerous articles criticizing the American corporations like Nestle, for example. Like "big pharma," a term I'd heard before, they were often referred to as, "big formula." I read an article from Stacker that discussed how the US doesn't regulate formula marketing, while many other countries do. The article said the US also didn't commit to the World Health Organization's globally accepted International Code of Marketing Breast-Milk Substitutes of 1981, which set standards for formula marketing. In 2020, the International Breastfeeding Journal found that large formula companies like Nestle or Abbott developed political relationships in Washington. Abbott has disclosed that they spent millions of dollars lobbying in Washington, according to the Stacker article. Data has shown that higher rates of breastfeeding correlate with nations' policies regarding mandatory parental leave. According to UNICEF, percentages of breastfed infants were the highest in East Asian countries and the lowest in

America. The world average for exclusively breastfed babies was 44% while it was 26% across North America.

It seemed to be a cultural choice of how long to continue. Most women receive glares or are the butt of jokes when they breastfeed for more than 6 months, yet the American Academy of Pediatrics (AAP) recommends continuing breastfeeding for at least the first two years. Even when women do wean their baby off breastmilk at one year, they still need to give them cow's milk to replace it. This seemed odd that breastmilk from another species was more socially acceptable for toddlers when my body was already making it and making it for a human.

I don't mean to bash moms who choose to formula feed. I'm grateful that we have technology and science these days that allow us the option. What I know from personal experience is that breastfeeding is fucking hard. Like pregnancy, it's a major physical and hormonal undertaking. I saw on TikTok that some women even develop a condition called D-MER, or Dysphoric Milk Ejection Reflex, where women experience intense feelings of dread when pumping. Some say nursing directly instead helps. The letdown reflex is triggered by Oxytocin and when the nipples are stimulated, it causes nerve impulses to the brain stem and hypothalamus that reduce dopamine. This process then allows for Prolactin, the milk hormone, to do its thing. The hormone drop and an imbalance somewhere in the process is believed to create the condition. It's known widespread among the motherhood community, yet it doesn't seem adequately studied. Many women suffer through D-MER thinking something is wrong with them since doctors never warn them of things like this, and it adds to the harrowing PPD experience.

Overall education regarding breastfeeding and how to support breastfeeding mothers seemed desperately needed among our species, especially in Western culture, and especially in the US.

40 Sleep Deprivation

Sleep deprivation is used as a war torture interrogation tactic for prisoners. It's internationally considered inhumane and often considered a war crime, yet new mothers take it on with little warning. You've probably heard the joking from parents, "Just wait until the baby comes for sleepless nights," they say with a chuckle. I wished instead they'd have grabbed my shoulders and shaken me into understanding the gravity. I thought I knew sleepless nights in my twenties. I'd spent a few all-nighters in the college library during finals or stayed out until the sun came up after taking too much molly at a concert. The difference was there was a finish line. In those days, I'd get to go to bed and nap away the morning. That wasn't sleep deprivation, it was just sleep *delay*. This time, there was no nap at the end of the tunnel. Postpartum was a state in which I needed rest more than ever before. I'd been through hell and back and had no idea I was about to experience this inhumane war crime for weeks. For three weeks, Claire slept only 10 minutes at a time.

One day, I was sitting on the couch in the living room with Claire breastfeeding at my chest. The dogs were locked in the office. I only knew it was daytime from the sunlight coming through the windows and because Connor was talking my ear off. He'd just gotten out of the shower and was standing next to me in a towel, wet and telling me some story about his work drama of the week. I shook my head, trying to listen and pay attention to him.

"Wait, you're dripping on the floor," I turned to scold him.

My heart sank when my eyes expected to meet his, but there was no one there. He had been so clearly there a second before.

"Connor?" I yelled, thinking maybe I just didn't see him walk back to the bathroom.

I looked at my phone. It was 11AM. He had texted, "I love you. How's it going so far today? I miss my girls!"

He wasn't home at all. He hadn't been home since 6AM even though I thought we had been talking for what felt like hours. He was a full-blown hallucinated apparition.

As time moved slowly over the next few weeks, days and nights melded together into one. I was awake for all of it. I saw every hour of the clock for days and days.

I'd frantically hit the buttons on my Amazon Fire Stick trying to turn down the loud obnoxious volume until, after a few minutes, I'd realize the TV was never even on. Months later, I'd found a page in my planner with illegible scribble. It almost looked like numbers, but they looked like I'd written them with my toes and my eyes closed. They squiggled and tilted drastically upward across the page. I remembered taking notes and writing phone numbers during a conversation with our Church's office secretary when I planned Claire's Baptism.

Carly apparently came to visit me a few days after we got home. She did the dishes in the sink and tidied the kitchen, knowing that I wouldn't be cleaning. I didn't even remember her being there, but apparently, we hung out for a few hours. I'm still grateful.

I only recall details from the first weeks of my postpartum era because I found an outlet in writing. While Claire fed, I'd use the blue light of my phone to stay awake. When mindlessly scrolling TikTok or online shopping made me drowsy, I started to journal in the Notes app about how I was feeling. It became cathartic. When I had no one to understand, I imagined writing to other women as the voice I wished I had to counsel me before embarking on the maternal voyage.

When people ask me the hardest part of pregnancy, birth, or postpartum, I immediately say the sleep deprivation and wished women and healthcare providers discussed this more. When I was off the painkillers after a few more weeks, I'd drive to the park and let us both sleep in the car for a few minutes, followed by a walk in nature. We spent our days in the backseat of my car at the park, breastfeeding, singing, sleeping, and writing in a sleep-deprived delirium. They're some of my favorite memories.

41 High Alert

When my friend Rachael got married several months later, I sat with a few of her Californian friends at a welcome brunch. They were all stunning and successful. In conversation, we learned that a few of us were moms. After a few glasses of champagne, we started to open up about how difficult it all was.

One of her friends, Kari, said that she struggled massively with postpartum psychosis and depression.

"I convinced myself that I gave my baby Drano," she recalled of her intense paranoia, a common symptom. I was so inspired by her candidness and told her that women need more of this honesty. She wasn't afraid that the other women at the table would think she was nuts.

"Medication saved my life," she told us. "Women can't be afraid to share anymore," she agreed.

Women are psychologically re-wired postpartum, and no one warns them of it. Amidst my sleep deprivation, I vented to some friends who'd had babies.

"Please tell me this gets better. I had no idea," I texted, feeling guilty for not reaching out to them more when they were postpartum.

"If you can, take a shower. I promise it really helps," my friend Khristee replied.

I remembered my reanimating shower in the hospital. "Shower" was a strong word for what occurred there. I stood half-slumped over while the hot water ran over my back, but it did restore some humanity in me. I did miss the vanilla and santal scents of my soaps and lotions. It was decided, like a big event. I waited all day for Connor to return from work. I let him settle in for a few minutes and assumptively asserted my goal.

"Connor I'm going to shower," I said confidently, "I need you to watch her for 20 minutes."

"Whoa what?" He backed away. "I have shit to do. I just got home, and I need to go to the gym now."

Typically, Claire was attached to me at all times with him just needing to change diapers in the evening if he was home. I thought about how for men and new fathers, "me time," included their hobbies, gym time, reading, video games, whatever they liked. For women and new mothers, "me time," or self-care included cleaning the house, cooking for the family, or personal hygiene. Suddenly, hygiene was an indulgence. I had to ask permission to take a shit, brush my teeth, or wash my body.

"Connor, you got to shower every day this week. I haven't showered in 4 days, please," I said.

"Okay fine, but please hurry so I can leave," he took the baby and kissed me on my greasy head.

I carefully stepped over the tub easing into the sting of my healing incision. I kept the lights bright, afraid that I'd fall asleep standing up and injure myself in the slippery shower. I let the warmth rain down over my tired and battered body. I felt each muscle relax in the heat and I took a deep breath of steam.

Abruptly, Claire screamed louder than usual over the rush of the water. It wasn't a hungry or tired-cry, it was hurt-cry. Something was wrong. As she screamed and screamed, with shampoo in my hair and tears in my eyes, I climbed my legs out of the tub and ran wet into the living room expecting a horrific scene. I was confused as I discovered Claire sleeping in Connor's arms, mouth open, dry eyes, with a relaxed brow. She hadn't been crying at all.

The look on Connor's face told me the horrific scene turned out to be me dripping wet suds on the hardwood floor, nude, bloody, and crazed.

I got back in the shower and the cries continued. I couldn't tell what was real.

"What's wrong? Is she crying?" I yelled over the water.

"No, Daddy's a pro. Your brain's broken again," Connor joked.

I couldn't enjoy the solace of the shower without the loud screeching cry that was somehow an aural hallucination.

I texted the other moms again, "Welp, I made it into that shower, but I think I've fully lost my marbles. I heard her crying the whole time, but it was all in my head."

"Oh yes, the phantom cries," Jacquleine replied. "I hate to tell you this, but they don't go away. I still have them." Her baby was 6 months older.

I googled "phantom cries" and learned it's another "common" and "normal" postpartum phenomenon. Blog posts and articles all detailed these hallucinations as being a fairly standard postpartum experience, yet they are not well-researched and rarely discussed.

"While we don't fully understand it, we do know having a baby changes the brain cells and neural connections in the mother's brain," one article quoting a UK pediatrician named Dr. Kiran Rahim read.

"Most parents are in a permanent state of stress in the early days, which wears the body down and places parents in a hyper alert state, perpetually ready to respond to even the slightest stress."

Intrusive Thoughts

Another tormenting mental postpartum phenomenon is the onslaught of vivid intrusive thoughts. "Intrusive thought" was a term I'd heard on TikTok as part of a silly meme cultured trend. Examples would be the sudden urge to stick your finger into candle wax, ruining the sheen of the surface, or the on-the-fly decision to order a third glass of wine. People used this term to describe trivial impulses. The videos about them were light and funny the way that people joke about "having OCD," when referring to keeping their room tidy, not realizing people who actually have OCD experience much darker twisted fears like needing to touch a doorknob ten times before leaving the house so their family won't die. The reality of intrusive thoughts postpartum similarly showed the over-use of these psychiatric terms.

Through the entire first year of motherhood, my mind interrupted every few hours with high-def disaster scenes. I'd be in a room with a staircase and see a vision of us tumbling down the stairs to a violent bloody end. I'd see my hot coffee sliding off the counter and scalding her, or the roof of my house suddenly collapsing. I'd pray feverishly for protection over our home from the trees outside from falling onto our house at just the right angle to crush us as we laid in bed. It was tough to concentrate on anything but these visual terrors and how my mind and body prepared for every final-destination-style scenario. Even 10 months later, I took deep breaths walking through the underground office parking garage as I envisioned the building crushing me, leaving Claire motherless. My logical mind knew they weren't real, but my nervous system did not. I learned that these intrusive thoughts are completely normal postpartum.

Common intrusive thoughts women report having include the baby suffocating, falling out of their arms or off the changing table, drowning, being burned, flying out of the car seat, or falling down the stairs.

Dr. Eynav Accort is listed as Director of the Cedars-Sinai Reproductive Psychology Program. I read an article from the Program's online blog. It said that about 70% of women experience them. Dr. Accord said that these intrusive thoughts are not harmful, and they're actually an evolutionary development that helps parents protect the baby by preparing for any disaster scenario.

Baby Blues

I'd heard that women cry a lot postpartum, and it's seen as endearing and silly. They call it the "baby blues." How cute! It seemed the line that separated things like "baby blues" and more serious life-threatening conditions like postpartum depression or psychosis were blurred. The common differentiator was the two-week mark. A sense of dooming, crushing depression, that we have this cutesy name for, is normal until it surpasses and worsens beyond two weeks. Medical professionals seemed to agree that's when it becomes more serious. Hormones, trauma, and increased anxiety all reshape a woman's mind drastically. According to The American College of Obstetricians & Gynecologists, maternal anxiety spikes postpartum any time in the first year, and/or during breastfeeding transitions, and/or her first returned menstrual cycle.

Many suffering women don't know there is support and treatment out there. Many lose their lives because of it.

At pediatrician appointments, I was asked on, in my opinion, oversimplified forms if I was feeling happy or sad or if I worried about my ability to care for my baby. Like most moms, I clicked "no." I lied because I was so afraid they'd take my baby from me. I knew I could take care of Claire. What I couldn't admit was that I couldn't take care of *me*.

Doctors often have new moms fill out the Edinburgh Postnatal Depression Scale. It asks simple questions like, "I have been able to laugh and see the funny side of things." The options range from "As much as I always could" to "not at all." Postpartum Depression is more nuanced than this. Women don't report a "happy or sad" type of experience. They may not recognize or feel connected to their baby, or they may even experience postpartum psychosis. Women need more than a questionnaire.

The Cedar Sinai blog was the first I'd seen of resources for women worried they may be experiencing a mental health crisis. A US government website, mchb.hrsa.gov lists 1-833-TLC-MAMA as a 24/7 phone or text line. It offers listening and referrals to local resources like support groups or healthcare providers. I couldn't believe this wasn't common knowledge among women who desperately need more proactive postpartum mental support. I'm grateful to have this opportunity to share it with you and only ask that you pass on the knowledge to other moms.

42 Postpartum Rage

I'd always been even-keel and could keep my cool even in the hottest water, another personality trait that seemed to have disappeared postpartum. The woman I knew so well, yet again, I didn't recognize. Every little thing lit my whole body on fire with anger. Connor and our dogs were usually the catalysts. Connor hadn't missed a beat. Nothing had changed for him during my pregnancy, and even now with my life and identity shattered, still, his life was the same. His time was his own. His body was his own. He had his hobbies and routines and meals and sleep. I was packed full of resentment, ready to burst of it at any moment.

The Cleveland Clinic says that Postpartum Rage and Postpartum Depression are different "but still closely related." Women experience outbursts of uncontrollable anger.

Yet again, no one warned me of this. I thought I was crazy.

One night, I was struggling to hold Claire and needed help as she cried, trying to latch onto my nipple. Just then, she leaked mustardy looking poop out of her diaper and all over me. I hadn't had a drink of water since yesterday and hadn't eaten anything but applesauce in more than 24 hours that I tried my best to keep down. It was about 3 weeks of being home, and I still had zero appetite. I knew I needed nutrients for breastfeeding, and I force-fed myself bread, applesauce, and a fistful of supplements every night to stay afloat; mostly a postnatal, magnesium, and Nutrafol to prevent my hair from falling out so much.

"Connor!" I yelled for help loudly enough for him to hear me, but softly enough to not scare Claire.

Expecting a response, I rather heard, "Where's our tank, guys!?" He was deep in a video game with his friends, stressed. My blood boiled and everything from my belly up to my forehead turned red hot. Holding Claire was the only safeguard preventing me from stomping in there and smashing the PC to bits.

"Connor!" I yelled louder. Still nothing. Enraged, heart pounding, I yelled a third time "CONNOR!!!!" Nothing. I growled like a wild animal, peeled myself off the couch in pain from my incision, holding onto Claire with her poop smeared all over both of us. I swung open the door, baby in one hand. With the other, I ripped his headset off his head as roughly as I could.

"You're done with this fucking headset," I snarled.

He looked up, startled, like a young boy whose game I'd interrupted with homework or bedtime. I looked at him with disgust, thinking he cared more about this virtual animated life than his real life. There was just as much gore and violence out here in my postpartum gloom as there was in their little pretend war game. Why wasn't it enough for him?

I was screaming at the top of my lungs, holding Claire's tiny ears shut. I'd never yelled at him or anyone like this before. I don't think he'd ever even heard me raise my voice. My eyes bulged, and I screamed each beastly insult, cutting as deeply as I could with my sleep deprived mind and reduced vocabulary.

"I'm out here caring for your baby alone, recovering from fucking surgery, haven't slept in weeks, the house is a fucking mess, and you're playing *video games* like an

immature child! Fucking grow up!" At least the word fuck
hadn't abandoned me like other pre-partum words had.

"I need your help, and you're in here like a loser!" I
could hear the other guys whispering on the headset. I
hoped they could hear me and receive the same insults.
They disgusted me too.

I was ready for battle. He just looked shocked. I scared
him. I felt like that Taylor Swift song, "Who's Afraid of
Little Old Me?" in which she, in a paranormal-level fury,
levitates down the street terrorizing the town. I thought the
level of my own postpartum bate would levitate me above
the streets of Pittsburgh to destroy the city like fucking
Godzilla with Claire hanging off my tit. I wasn't prepared
for such rage and hatred of someone I loved so much. Still,
I needed him.

"Okay, okay," he said softly. He took Claire and started
to clean us both off as I reduced to tears into his chest.

43 Childcare

I held Claire close to my chest stroking her hair behind her ear as I breastfed her in the dark. I couldn't believe how big she'd gotten, but also how small she still was. How could I leave a baby this small? It was 3AM, but I didn't miss sleep this time. I needed every minute with her because we only had a few more days left until the eminent cataclysm. Maternity leave was ending soon. The hardest, yet truly happiest and most fulfilling time I'd ever known in my entire life was ending. I can only describe the feeling of losing it as doom, panic, and heartbreak.

I kept my tired eyes open during these overnight feeds by journaling in my notes app. Maybe I'd write a book one day. Nobody told me, but I'll tell them, I thought. When I was too tired to form coherent thoughts, I scrolled on TikTok. The blue light of my phone hypnotized me as Claire suckled, and I fell deep into rabbit holes about the emotional damage fulltime daycare imposes on babies under three.

Daycare

There are conflicting studies that all seemed to lack the newer reality of daycare for our generation's babies, which was that children no longer start at age 3-4. In previous generations, the smaller population of kids who were even in daycare began closer to school age, and it was only for a few hours a day or 1-3 days a week. In the US, some called it "pre-school." Now, many start when they are only weeks old, a critical time for physical and emotional development to be attached to their mother. They're there longer than an adult work shift or a big kid's school day, to account for both their mom's shift and commutes there and back. Claire would need to be there 50+ hours a week, even as I snuck out the office door a few minutes early.

These forceful separations of mother and baby and their effects are somewhat uncharted. I read the findings of the INCHD Study of Early Child Care and Youth Development. It began in the 90s and continued to follow children years later to assess their emotional and behavioral patterns. It found that at about a year old, more time spent in daycare was associated with an increased risk for insecure infant-mother attachment relationship. When they grew closer to school age, they struggled with social competence and behavioral issues and negative peer play. The study seemed to have solid controls and included several demographics that accounted for things like family income, infant temperament, and maternal education. The findings looked clear. As they grew older, cumulative daycare time predicted things like substance abuse and behavioral struggles into adolescence. I wanted to poke holes in the research for my own comfort, but I couldn't find any.

Triggering Research

I came across Erica Komisar on clips from numerous popular podcasts. I'm sure I've already triggered some of you with this name. She triggers me too. She polarizes moms. I'm not here to argue about which conflicting beliefs mean more. I just wanted to straighten out what's best for my baby, just like you are, even if I knew I couldn't deliver it. According to her website, Komisar has been in clinical social work and psychology for 40 years and has written about the first three years of a child's life. She writes about the biological and psychological importance of a baby's attachment to their mother during this time. She's critical of the lack of maternity leave in the US. This triggers and upsets moms like me who, in a storm of crippling guilt cry out,

"Easy for you to say! I don't *want* to leave my baby. I MUST!"

I challenged myself to listen even when it hurt my chest to hear the facts. The reality seemed to be that the modern American system for motherhood contradicts what's best for babies in the first three years of life. Separation early in infanthood does affect them. If we can't admit this together, how will we ever push for a change in things like more humane maternity leave policy?
My take is that if we want to continue to work fulltime, we do need to address the uncomfortable facts (even when they piss us off and crush our hearts) and use them to create more family-supportive work environments.

What about big kids?

Even after the baby stages, my heart broke differently when I thought of Claire being a bit bigger at daycare.

"What will we do with her in the Summers when she's school-age?" I asked Connor, rhetorically. I knew he, like most of our generation pre-parenthood, didn't realize that daycare stops at age 5 when kids begin school.

"She'll be at the pool everyday like we were!" he said excitedly, remembering childhood memories at the playground or public pools with his friends.

"We'll be at work. We'll sometimes get to do that stuff on Saturdays or Sundays, but she won't get a summer break," I said with wet eyes.

"Oh shit. That's right. Kids don't really get summer breaks anymore then, do they? Unless they have a stay-at-home-parent or fulltime nanny? Who can fucking afford those anyway," he said.

Aside from the sadness, there isn't a clear answer for what happens when kids are in the in-between era, when they're too old for daycare yet too young to be on their own all day at home. We'd have to hire a fulltime nanny, and local nanny annual salaries ranged from $70-$85K. My own base salary was $65K. Yes, sometimes there are summer camps or programs at churches like "vacation Bible school." Trust me, I've looked. Those are only a few hours a day and usually only last a few weeks. Nothing like that would cover the 50+ hours of our fulltime work week and commutes.

The Girl Boss Scam

Since pre-school, as long as I can remember, the goal was always to get a high-paying full-time job. Why else did I work so hard to get into college? This was simply what was expected of my generation of "girl bosses." In first grade, we mastered corporate technology like Microsoft Excel or PowerPoint. Going to college and getting the fancy job was the only real option ingrained in us from the start. So, what happens when the "girl boss" gets pregnant? Everything I'd known and worked for in life had turned out to be some sort of sick joke. I was supposed to work hard from pre-school through college to get this glorious fulltime job and career. Feminists fought for my rights and freedom for decades. For what? This? This couldn't be what they had in mind.

I thought back to the dinner conversation with friends where they talked about how their companies discarded pregnant women. I hated that I understood why companies wanted to toss us like used garbage. I couldn't perform as well while pregnant. Now that I'd be going back to work, I'd need the rest of the staff and my clients to accommodate for me coming in late due to daycare-drop-off. I'd need to leave sometimes to take Claire to the pediatrician, and I'd be so sleep-deprived and forgetful that even I had to admit I was no longer a star employee. I needed a new flexibility that I didn't feel safe enough to ask for in the corporate world.

The only heartbreak I'd felt that even came close to this was when my mother died. It was paralyzing grief. The loving stay-at-home mother I'd always dreamed of being and embodied these last 14 weeks was dying, to be buried next to the other beloved versions of me I'd already lost this year.

I saw some women posting mid-cry in their cars on TikTok.

"Our country gives at least two years of maternity leave. No way the US doesn't mandate any at all. I don't believe that." Comment sections with replies like these seared through me.

It was so inhumane that people from other nations didn't even believe it. This couldn't be part of this "American Dream." Fierce guilt drove me into fight or flight. I cannot physically separate from her for 11 hours a day. I just can't, I thought. She was only 12 weeks old and relied on me so heavily. I hated Connor for not being rich, hated the lack of US societal support, and hated myself for getting us into this mess.

"I'll never forgive myself for this," I declared internally as my tears fell on Claire's cheek. I hearted a TikTok comment that said, "Working women in America… what a fucking scam."

Cataclysm

I didn't truly think I had the big official Postpartum Depression. I didn't recognize how far I'd fallen, and I didn't know to seek professional help. If this resonates, please do.

My heartache grew dark, fluxing between panic, ennui, and rage. I looked ahead at my life and hated what I saw. I hated that I'd break my connection with this baby to force myself to the office all day every day and only get an hour or less in the evening to be the new real me, her mother. Would she even know me? I felt stuck. This was my only option, and I didn't want it, so I didn't want to live anymore. I concluded life wasn't worth this pain of tearing apart mother and infant. I imagined all the soft ways I could end it. I decided swallowing a bunch of pills seemed the least violent, least painful, and most considerate way for Connor to find my body without mess or gore. I handwrote a note for him on my nightstand with instructions and passwords for our utilities and finances. I'd take the pills while he held Claire downstairs, thinking that I just needed a nap upstairs. I'd leave my body tucked into my bed, peaceful. I constructed the whole plan for hours while I breastfed Claire. I looked down at her and stopped, whipped back to reality like the reverb of a snapping rubber band, sucked in by the inertia of my love for her, the agape.

It rescued me every time. The only thing that kept me from taking my own life postpartum was knowing Claire was here.

And so, I stayed.

44 Daycare

On the Friday before my first Monday back to work, the daycare allowed us to do a "practice day." We'd drop Claire off for a couple of hours to get used to being there before she'd spend 50 hours a week there. We'd go from spending nearly every minute together to nearly every waking minute apart. I barely trusted Connor to babysit her when I'd go to the store. I had no clue how to leave her with a room full of strangers and germs every day in perpetuity.

"Let's do a lunch date so we don't think about it," Connor suggested. "We can drink." We decided on an Italian restaurant connected to my office building.

"We'll drop Claire off and practice the drive downtown for you," he said, wrapping his arms around Claire and me as she slept on my chest. We swayed back and forth as a unit, and he kissed my head, sensing my impending breakdown.

"Plus, that means you have to drive, and I can be passenger princess." He let an evil laugh, and I rolled my eyes and smiled.

I cried during the whole lunch into a martini and only lasted 45 minutes.

"We're so lucky we even got into this place," Connor said as we packed her bag together.

He was right. I'd never heard of the daycare shortages and waitlists until my HR rep asked how many waitlists I'd made it onto so far.

"I'm only 3 months pregnant," I told her.

"Oh honey. Hang up this call right now and hit the phones," she warned me.

"Hi, I'm pregnant and calling to see if you have any openings this Fall for an infant?" I asked repeatedly.

With babies and kids crying in the background, I'd be met with a laugh and, "We have a five-year waitlist. What's your email address? We'll add you."

After dozens of calls, I finally made it on two waitlists and prayed daily one would call back. About a month before I went back to work, my phone rang.

"We had a spot open up in the infant room unexpectedly," the director said. "The family moved out of state. This is first-come-first-serve with the waitlist, and whoever gets here quickest can have the spot."

"Sign us up. What do you need?"

"If you can be here tomorrow at noon with a $500 deposit, it's yours."

On Monday I walked into the nursery room at the daycare, greeted by three of her teachers. Ms. Mary was clearly in charge with her clipboard and iPad. There were 12 babies total in the room. The legal limit in PA was four infants to each adult. Ms. Lisa sat in a rocking armchair bottle-feeding one baby boy in her arms and using both of her feet to bounce two baby girls in their seats on the floor. Another baby cried half-asleep next to her in an electric swing. Ms. Marsha was gently jerking two of the wheeled cribs as two more boys drifted to sleep.

"Hi Claire!" Ms. Marsha approached me, ready to hold her, but she kept her distance until I was ready. I restrained my cries as softly as I could and kissed her cheeks and head over and over before handing her off into this stranger's arms. My baby's life and innocence were at this person's mercy, and I didn't know even know them.

I passed her bag to Ms. Mary. I'd packed her bottles, favorite blanket, extra onesies, diapers, frozen bags of breastmilk, and formula. I couldn't over-produce enough milk to have a surplus to send to daycare, so we had to start combo-feeding.

"She ate 30 minutes ago." I said with a huge lump in my throat without taking my eyes off Claire. I wanted to snatch her back and say, "FUCK YOU ALL," running up the wooded hillside I could see outside the window, never to return. They'd never find me, I thought. Instead, I just sobbed.

"She has sensitive skin, so we use liniment and cotton pads instead of baby wipes," I reminded them. "They're all in her bag."

I'd learned in all this baby research that diaper rashes seem to be uncommon in other countries. In France, they use an olive oil-based product, liniment, to clean the babies' bums, and diaper rashes aren't common at all, whereas in the US, they are routine. I vowed to save Claire from the chemicals and can proudly confirm we avoided diaper rash, minus one week when she had diarrhea from a daycare stomach bug.

"She and you will both adjust," Ms. Mary said. "We'll take good care of her."

I drove in silence through the route Connor practiced with me. I thought again about killing myself at the red light ahead of the Liberty Bridge above the river. I could just drive right off into the water and end this pain, I thought. Quickly, I remembered my phobia of deep waters, and the green light sucked me back to reality.

"You'll be okay. I love you. I miss her too," Connor texted. I didn't respond. He went to work daily and hadn't been connected to her body and soul the way I had. I was grieving. My stomach hurt the way it did when I'd grieved my mother's death, and I couldn't eat.

Back to work

"Pull it together, Katie," I told myself out loud through sniffles and heaves. I aggressively wiped tears off my cheeks to preserve my mascara and concealer looking in my little fold-down car mirror. I'd made it to the parking garage. All I could think about was how far away I was from Claire. I fought off every instinct to get closer to her as fast as I physically could. I fumbled around my bag in my passenger seat. I was already late. I didn't give a flying fuck. It's not possible to do daycare drop-off and still make it to the office in time for business hours.

"My breast pump machine, the weird long tubes connected to it, the power cord, the milk bags, my laptop, my building security badge, my wallet, my phone…okay," I said aloud, confirming the necessary inventory for the day ahead.

I felt the familiar click-clack… click-clack of my heels on the matte marble floor of the office building. I kept my head down and beelined for the elevator to the 20th floor. On the way up, I noticed my reflection in the mirrored elevator walls and remembered the similar mirrored elevator in New York on my birthday trip almost exactly a year ago. I saw two starkly different reflections as I grieved that woman, that version of me, who died just 14 weeks ago. She'd know what to do and how to handle this day. I made eye contact with this new and strange reflection. My skin looked gray and my dark eye circles showed through my layers of concealer. I got about 2 hours of sleep the night prior. That was actually pretty good. Claire was entering another sleep regression, and I accepted that working while sleep deprived would be the new norm.

"Sleep while the baby sleeps!" This is what generations of women have been told. It doesn't work anymore. I'd be at work while Claire naps.

I forced myself to turn off my emotion like one of the characters in *The Vampire Diaries* series. It's a cheesy vampire show I used to watch every Halloween season. The vampires could focus and switch off their "humanity," so they wouldn't feel a thing. No guilt or sadness. I fought every cell of me wanting to throw my bag, run for my life back to the car, speed back to daycare, snatch Claire into my arms and drive until no one could ever find us. Both my body and soul begged me to do it. With every step, I almost did.

My boobs hurt. I was grateful that I got to pump soon. The bright, loud office offended my senses. I'd grown accustomed to dimmed light and quiet moments with Claire, comfy in my bed learning about each other. A slow life. Instead, the glass walls of the conference room vibrated with the bass of some rap song they were blasting in the morning to wake everyone up. I squinted at the fluorescent lights and noticed through the windowed walls that the sun wasn't up yet.

My friend Hannah gasped as I turned the corner into the office kitchen. "Katieeeeeee oh my gosh it's so good to see you! Welcome back!" She hugged me.

A few others heard her and ran over to do the same. They had no idea how badly I'd needed the human warmth, but I knew none of them could understand.

"It's good to be back," I lied through my teeth.

I was a fraud cosplaying as the old me. She was dead, and only I knew it. I was there. I'd held her hand while she died, slowly over the course of 10 months like a terminally ill patient, and finally disappeared, but no one else realized it or if they did, they didn't care to mourn her. I grieved her privately in secret. They didn't know this new me.

The other Katie, the dead one, would have spent an hour getting ready that morning. She'd arrive early at 7:15AM EST to get a head start on the day with a cappuccino in hand. She cared about doing a good job. She'd wear a sleek outfit. A sharp blouse with pointed-toe heels and a blazer to show she meant business. Clients always took her more seriously in a blazer, a weird puzzle piece in the psychological game of sales. This new me turned out to be a bad actress. I'd shown up with dirty hair. When would I have time to wash it these days? Would I *ever* wash my hair again, and take 15 minutes in the shower away from the precious 45 minutes I have left daily with Claire? Hell no. Permanently greasy hair was a fine price to pay.

My face flushed as I noticed I'd lactated all over my sage green satin blouse. My leg hair peeked out of the bottom of my pants. The heels were old Katie's everyday shoes. I felt wrong wearing them, like wearing the shoes of a dead woman, almost disrespectful.

The office seating arrangement was different, and I realized they'd packed up my belongings, and I no longer had a seat. I really did die, and they'd packed up my stuff and moved on without me.

"Does anyone know where the box of my stuff is?" I yelled into the office.

"Um… maybe check the supply closet?" someone yelled over the sea of monitors.

I sifted through books and supplies that weren't mine and pieced out each thing that was. I remember this jacket,

I thought. This emergency deodorant, dry shampoo, pink
Post-its. It was strange, the same way we sort through
belongings of a loved one after they've passed. Each
mundane meaningless item suddenly evokes emotion and
memories of that person. For example, my mother used to
wash her face with Ponds, the one with the blue cap. I
never noticed the smell, but now that she's gone, the
cream's powdery scent stops me in my tracks. Here was all
my stuff, as if I'd just walked away one day from my desk
and never came back. That same woman never would. My
tears hit my knees, but I shook my head clear of emotion. I
left the supply closet with a neutral half-smile I'd wear like
a Halloween mask for the next 6 months.

45 Pumping

The office was huge and modern, very millennial or gen z corporate style as far as the interior design. It has industrial-chic concrete floors and sleek glass-walled conference rooms with a themed mural on each wall. The desks are Agile, open-concept. We each have our own desk and work-station, but there are no cubicles. It's loud and lively. Recent renovations also included a small, unlabeled room near the kitchen. It had a counter with a mini-fridge and a little sink, a chair, and a mirror.

"This is the Mothers Room," the renovation project manager told us on the first day it opened. "If and when someone becomes a mother, this will be for them to pump breastmilk in while they're in the office."

For years, we never had anyone become a mother, so it became a multi-purpose extra conference room of sorts. It's also where Cintas hung the first-aid supplies and medications like Advil and Tylenol or cough drops. Heading back to work, I hoped people would remember its original intended purpose.

I sent a people-pleasing message to the office's Teams Chat.

"Hey guys! So excited to be back. I know we all use the Mothers Room for meetings and whatnot, but I'll need to be in there for a while a few times a day. If we can refrain from using it at 8:00, 10:00, 12:00, 2:00, and 4:00 I'd so appreciate it! I can be flexible if you really need the room, just message me and I'll adjust!"

My friends emphasized the message and sent hearts to the chat, but every day, the room was often full. At least once a day, I sat outside of it with engorged and dripping breasts. I was too uncomfortable to knock and reference my uncontrollable bodily fluids. I was lucky enough to work for a company that has such a room at all. Most women in the US pump in the bathrooms or their car, lacking sanitation, privacy, and dignity.

I was used to nursing Claire at home, comfortably topless, skin to skin. Her warm little body attached to mine like a puzzle piece I'd always been missing. Both she and I wanted to do nothing else all day but nurse and stare at each other enchanted, spellbound, intoxicated by Oxytocin coursing through us. This is not only the setting that felt emotionally important, but medically, Oxytocin and low stress levels are what prompt the body to produce milk. The baby's saliva also physically sends the message to the body to concoct a perfect custom recipe her body needed that day. The plastic of the pump wouldn't offer the same customization.

As the lock to the Mothers Room clicked for the first time, I dabbed the tears as quickly as I could to prevent the makeup from running and compromising my disguise. Claire was part of me, body and soul, and we were miles away from each other. I went from our warm love bubble of nursing to a cold, sterile, corporate room with fluorescent lights and the murmur of meetings in surrounding conference rooms. The love bubble had turned into a Cortisol cloud. I attached the pump and turned on the motor. It hurt a bit and never felt like the right angle or size. For twenty minutes, this machine tugged on me as I cried and did my best to keep up with the familiar onslaught of emails and messages. Milk barely came out unless I stared at pictures of her to trick my body.

"I'm in here… Sorry!" I said to knocks on the door. Every 10 minutes or so, the doorknob would wiggle.

I'd hear, "Ugh I need to get in there. I need an Advil." Or "Hi, I'm with Cintas and I'm here to replenish the office supplies in there. How long will you be?"

Breastfeeding felt so private, like going to the restroom, yet I felt exposed and imposing on a multipurpose supply closet.

46 Mothership to Partnership

Motherhood forced me to let go of Connor's hand and allow him to tread water on his own. It forced us, trial by fire, to become a different couple. I didn't realize how much I was mothering him all these years until I no longer had bandwidth to do so. I loved him and felt guilty that I wasn't the girl he found years ago.

It reminded me of the movie *"Night Bitch."* It was a weird film following a mother as she became a werewolf-like animal. A woman with a once blossoming career, a fiery personality with a clear and respected place in society, and a strong identity, had now become a fulltime mother and household manager, broken down by exhaustion. She and her husband resent each other. He feels alone in the relationship without the hot young girl he signed up for. She resents him because she shoulders the burdens of motherhood in ways men can't and handles the household mental load.

In one scene, her husband yells, "What happened to the girl I married? What happened to the girl that inspired me and made me challenge this world in new and interesting ways? What happened to my wife?"

She looked at him, incredulously. "She died in childbirth."

My relationship with Connor in our first year of parenthood radically changed. A book called *"The Motherload"* by Sarah Hoover about her postpartum depression came out when I was about 5 months postpartum. We had very different experiences in our initiation into motherhood. She lived in NYC, was married to a cool rich artist, and had a night-nanny. I was jealous. Still, I loved her brutal honesty and related to the way she spoke about her marriage.

She said, "Motherhood made me stop mothering my husband."

I noticed the same in my own relationship. When I released control, or had it ripped from my hands, he had no choice but to take the reins.

6-Week Milestone

The 6-week gyno appointment is long-awaited by husbands because it's when women are medically cleared for activity, including sex. Doctors specializing in pelvic floor health argue that it should be much longer.

"Your abs have healed back together," the midwife said pressing over my still sensitive belly. I was relieved because, since I didn't get my 2-week appointment, I was worried she'd tell me I was dying.

"Your incision looks great too." It didn't look great to me. It was red and scabby and reminded me of the trauma of being gutted on a table. It was surrounded with stretchmarks, all encompassed by a new flabby pouch of fat and stretched skin. I thought I'd never feel pretty again.

"Are you interested in birth control?" she asked.

"No, thank you." I couldn't imagine ever having sex again. I was terrified of doing this again, but somehow more terrified of Connor. I was so disconnected and resented him so deeply that being intimate felt fraudulent. I didn't want to be touched. I was so overstimulated and over-touched at all times that, the moment Claire napped, I just wanted to shower or feed myself.

"Well… are we good?" Connor asked, excited on the drive home and touching my upper thigh. I remembered the times he'd fingered me in the car. We used to be so connected and had so much fun as a couple. That version of us felt so far away.

"Yep," I said in a fake pleasant tone, dreading the inevitable.

We tried the next day in the shower. I was so scared. He took off his shorts, and I didn't recognize his body anymore. He may as well have unsheathed a knife. It hurt the way it did when I lost my virginity, and I cried afterward. I wanted to get it over with. My body felt like it belonged to everyone but me. It got better over time and started to feel good again after a few weeks, but I wasn't emotionally prepared for the feelings of triggered trauma and violation it stirred up the first few times. I worried our relationship wouldn't weather the storm.

Slowly, Connor had to accept that I could no longer manage the household, breastfeed, work fulltime, and be a sex nymph in my spare-time (I had none).

The villain?

I probably have inadvertently painted Connor a villain in this story, but he's not. Men aren't educated on the intensity of having a baby. They see the expectations that women will be back to work a week after birth and hear women say how lovely the whole experience has been. How could he have known if even *I* didn't?

When we bought a new house 8 months later, I noticed he was changed too. He barely touched his godforsaken video games anymore. That alone turned me on. He worked 7 days a week and had career goals with higher stakes as a father with a family depending on him. He moved all our furniture and facilitated our entire relocation while I focused on Claire and my work.

When I came home from shifts, he had Claire home with a clean diaper and dinner sizzling on the stove. I'd drop my heavy purse, kick off my heels, relieved and greeted with a big hug from both of them.

Our new version of us certainly wasn't perfect, but I released the stiff control I had in the beginning of our relationship, and I felt the comfort of a true partner for the first time. I loved him differently. We were soul-tied in a way I could have never imagined with any other man. By now, he'd seen every part of me I'd hidden from others. He knew my stretchmarks and my scarred skin. I wouldn't even fart in front of him a year ago for fear he'd realize that girls don't shit glitter and sunshine. Now, he'd wiped blood from my ass and picked me up off the toilet in the hospital, yet he still wanted me. He'd seen beneath my masks, yet there he was reaching for me. He was still in love with me after seeing the cruddiest, stickiest, hateful parts of me. No one had seen me truly naked the way Connor now had. This new love was tender and safe. Parenthood had changed him and us too.

47 New & Employed Mother

When it comes to being a working mom, I wish I could offer you a clean ending in which I cracked the code of how to bilocate like a Catholic Saint and be both the fiery girl boss at work and the present mom at home. I wish it were true that women can do it all, but it's not. I can offer that motherhood untied a knot I'd created between my work performance and my survival. Before pregnancy, it was end of the world every time I disappointed a client or we lost budget for a project. It was a release to have something more important to me than work. It wasn't that I didn't care about my work anymore. In many ways, I cared more deeply with higher stakes and a family to support. I had a baby to care for and a mortgage to pay. There is now *more* to life than the daily grind. My self-worth is no longer tied to performance. I knew it before, but now I could *feel* it.

The challenge is that us moms are split in two every day. Part of me is motivated to contribute to our growing household, and the other aches to be with Claire at every second. I watched influencers like Pookie and Jet witness their new baby's milestones like sitting up for the first time or standing in her crib, or crawling. I felt (and still feel) jealous that I can't witness these things with Claire. These are moments that, to non-parents, sound mundane, but are the greatest wonders for parents. I watched most of these through the daycare app. For example, they told me how hard she'd been practicing standing in her crib after nap time. Finally, one day my phone beeped. Ms. Mary sent me a photo of Claire standing up with proud straight legs and her hands gripping the wooden edges. The look on her face was pure accomplishment. Her eyes were locked with Ms. Mary's behind the camera, and I wished she looked to me in these moments instead. I thought back to the *Sex & The City* scene when Miranda's stuck at work night and day, and her baby grows more attached to her nanny and housekeeper, Magda than he is to her. In one scene, she's finally home with him and he cries and cries.

She's holding him desperately and says to her friends, "Don't worry. He just misses his mommy…Magda."

As a fulltime working mom, I don't get to make many decisions for my own baby. We follow what the daycare requires. I'm usually not sure what she eats for breakfast or snacks, but I do pack her lunch. I don't know what they're teaching her or what methods they're using, if any, to develop her brain. I don't know what values they're instilling in her.

A young coworker asked me, "Have you been teaching her sign language? I think I want to do that when I have a baby one day!"

"I only get 45 minutes with her each day, aside from the weekend," I reluctantly told her. "So, I don't really get the time to do those things, but I'd love to if I didn't work!"

"45 minutes?!" She was shocked, and so were the other girls around her. I was in their shoes before I got pregnant. My instinct was to lie to them, like women did with me years ago, but I forced myself to be honest.

"We work the full day, and just like you, I have a 40-minute commute home. She goes to bed about 45 minutes later, and I have to use that time to make her dinner." I hated saying it all out loud, but I thought these girls ought to know the truth of what they were in for. You should too.

I do my best to make the most of the little time I get with my daughter. I eliminate the time I'd waste at the grocery store by ordering it to be delivered through an app called Instacart. I have diapers arrive on a monthly subscription, and even have fresh organic meals delivered every other week so that I don't need to cook as often. Find these tweaks in your own schedule and prepare.

So, now what?

Now that you too know what women commonly endure in pregnancy and postpartum, we can now have an educated conversation on what they *need*. Firstly, legislation, especially in the US. American families deserve humane maternity leave and healthcare backed by medical research so that women can do what's best for their bodies and their babies. This benefits companies too. Women can perform more efficiently if they're alive, healthy, well-rested, and well-supported. Dads need paternity leave too. The US needs to catch up to the rest of global society in this area, and fast.

In the workplace, flexibility is key. The year I came back from having my baby was not just the hardest year I'd ever experienced. It also ended up being the year my performance and success sky-rocketed. I hit all-time-highs in client revenue and performance metrics, I got promoted to a management position, and I wrote this book. I credit my ability to reach these professional heights to my partnership with my manager, Ella. I owe this success to her. She knew I could perform and bring my whole self to work each day if I had flexibility and the expectation that the workday wouldn't be perfect. She'd cover for me while I ran to the daycare for things like a Mother's Day Brunch

and tell me not to stress if I needed to pick her up early
when she was sick. She knew that my workday and
business hours would also now be more fluid. Through
over-communication on my part and understanding on hers,
we made it work. After daycare drop-off, I got to work late
at 8:30AM each day. In order to ensure I got to see Claire
for dinner before she went to bed, I took my last calls of the
day from my car and left at 4:45PM. It was fewer hours
than I technically was supposed to work. I worked from
home at least once a week, and more if Claire was sick or
going through a sleep regression. And guess what,
corporate world? The world kept fucking spinning, and
with the relief of the pressure and rigidity we usually place
on working moms, I was able to perform at an even *higher*
level.

I urge you to be honest in conversations about what
you're experiencing with your healthcare providers, your
partner, your friends, and your employer. I hope that you
aren't afraid to share details, and I hope you demand what
you need.

48 New Home

When Claire was almost a year old, I was working from home while she was at daycare. On my lunch break, it was finally quiet. I thought I ought to clean. I scanned my living room that once was immaculately tidy. Just two years ago everything was so different in that old life I'd mourned this year. Back then, the beige couch complimented the white woodworking, fresh white hydrangeas were neatly arranged in a vase on the mantle. The décor was chicly neutral. I smiled at the now loud primary colors of the children's books that were far from aesthetically chic. Red, green, and blue clashed all over my bookcases. A big stuffed Mickey Mouse our neighbor bought her laid in a pile of pink toys in her playpen in the corner. Everything had animals on it in some form, and instead of the neutral artwork that once hung on the wall, I instead faced a penguin and cardinal made of construction paper and cutouts of her hands that her daycare teachers made with her. These were more precious than anything in the Louvre. I looked to the dining room. The fine China and crystal chandelier were now outshined by a pink plastic high-chair and a pile of unfolded baby laundry. Tiny onesies, a sleep sack, soft and small wash-clothes, and a flamingo hooded towel. Old me would have hated this scene, but she didn't exist anymore. Thank God. No interior designer could create a home for me as beautiful as this. It was perfect. I didn't want to change a single detail, and I never wanted to leave this stage of life.

Motherhood stopped me dead in my tracks and killed me, or at least my former identity. It brought into this world

instead a woman changed. I now clung to the hands of time
to try desperately to pry them backward to a screeching
halt. I cried holding her pink bunny she'd left on the couch.
I imagined how my house would look neutral, clean and
tidy once again because, one day, there would be no tiny
laundry on the dining room table and no animal themed
crafts made out of her little hands coming home each
month. I'd be well-rested and sleep in on the weekends
again. I'd eat a warm dinner in peace again. I'd go on trips
without being so devastatingly missed. My body would feel
my own. This was what I thought I wanted and what I'd
grieved postpartum. I now realized I'd get it all back, yet I
didn't want it. I couldn't imagine a life without my baby.
She'd be replaced by a grownup one day, whom I'd love
just as much, I'm sure, yet differently. These little hands
and feet, these giggles, and two tiny teeth would be gone.
I'd have the privilege of knowing this little girl for such a
short time and then grieve her with each new phase all over
again. In fact, it would one day be my job to help her pack
up this life and leave me here to mourn it alone in my tidy
house. I realized this was the true feeling of home. I
thought it was this house and its historic connection to my
past. We'd just bought a new house and were moving soon.
I wasn't as sad as I imagined I'd be. All my true pieces of
home would be coming with me.

Heaven on Earth

I kept a list in my phone called "Dinner Table
Questions" I'd curated over the course of several years, and
I'd only pull it out at the dinner table when the vibe felt
right. Friends asked for the list constantly, and I'd joke,
"No it's sacred!" It launched us into conversations of

debate, laughs, or tears. The questions ranged from gross "would you rathers" to existential crisis or moral dilemma. My favorite question to ask, though, was one that often lets you peer into the hearts of those at the table. It works best after two bottles of wine, dessert, and dimmed lights when everyone has their guard down. It goes, "You just died. You meet God. He grants you five more minutes on earth to experience something one last time. Where do you go?" People usually take it to painstaking detail down to the drink in their hand and the song playing in the background. It's often someone's favorite concert that rocked them full of adrenaline or swinging on the childhood swingset, hiking in some exotic mountain range. My boss' boss said his was in a hammock swing at his grandparents home in wine country California. When I first starting dating Connor, he said his was at a music festival in his early twenties in New York City with his closest friends.

I never knew what to say for my own.

I thought back on this question, and my answer was easy now. God must know my order exactly already. I pray he'll have it ready for me when I've left this earth in an elderly state after a long life. I'd want to be two months postpartum in my childhood home's messy bedroom, sleep deprived and still healing. It's 3AM, dark and quiet as if we're the only ones awake in the world, an intimacy nothing else replicates. Connor's sound asleep to my left. His face is young again. He looks strong and healthy with his hair still brown and red, just the way I'd remember him. The only song playing is my own soft and strained voice. It's young again too and singing a slowed and probably off-key version of "My Girl" by the Temptations. I look down at my hand and no longer see wrinkles and age spots, but instead my smooth young fingers stroke a tiny peaceful face. Claire is nestled in my left arm, drinking from me. There she is. She's so small again. Her hair is still dark brown before it turned blonde and grew to her shoulders. Her skin is soft and so fair it's transparent and pink. I can hear her exhaling little swallow sounds. I nuzzle my nose into her fine brown hair and inhale her newborn baby smell. I imagined thanking God for this last taste of Heaven on earth and welcoming death, as I once thought this was the nadir of my life. I now realize, it was the precious summit.

Acknowledgements

Thank you to my editor, Becky Alexander, who both perfected this work and encouraged me to keep going.

Thank you to my cover design artist, Rachael Hendrix, a generation talent with unparalleled vision and skill, and a dear friend.

Thank you to my publicist, Elena Jones, for spreading the message to wider audience of women.

Thank you to Connor, for sticking by my side throughout my mothership voyage and saving it from sinking everyday.

Thank you to Claire. You are everything to me, and I couldn't imagine being anything else in this universe other than your mom.

Thank you to my mom, Terri. Motherhood unveils a woman's own mother in a new light, and I see it all now. You were the supreme example of maternal love and warmth I dream to achieve.